PRESCRIBING LIFESTYLE

A Doctor's Prescription for Lasting
Weight Loss and Vibrant Health

Dr Avi Charlton

First published by Ultimate World Publishing 2025
Copyright © 2025 Dr Avi Charlton

ISBN

Paperback: 978-1-923425-79-8
Ebook: 978-1-923425-80-4

Cover design: Ultimate World Publishing
Layout and typesetting: Ultimate World Publishing
Editor: Alex Floyd-Douglass

Ultimate World Publishing
Diamond Creek,
Victoria Australia 3089
www.writeabook.com.au

ULTIMATE WORLD
— PUBLISHING —

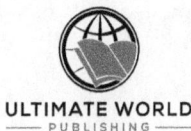

TESTIMONIALS

———————— ◆◇◆ ————————

"Dr Avi Charlton is an inspirational lifestyle doctor, focusing on holistic strategies and a low-carb way of eating. She walks her talk, constantly challenging herself, growing, learning, and always reaching for more knowledge and achievement in her life. I am so grateful to be able to call her both a friend and a colleague.

Avi's latest achievement is to write a book, in which she prescribes a lifestyle for health and weight loss. Avi guides you through the lifestyle pillars of nutrition, exercise, sleep, stress management, community support, and managing addictions. It is filled with a balance of science and real-life experiences, as well as simple, actionable steps you can take to be healthier and happier. If you are open to unlearning old habits, discovering the truth about nutrition, and are willing to take control of your health, this is the book for you. I urge you to read it… It might just change your life!"

Carla Veith-Carter,
Founder of *Keto By Design*

"Dr Avi Charlton is not only one of my most respected business associates, but also someone I now have the privilege of calling a dear friend. What sets her apart is her genuine desire to offer wellness advice across a wide range of topics, especially those that everyday people often struggle with in silence. She approaches her work not just with professionalism, but with a rare authenticity and compassion that radiates through every interaction. Her heart is truly in the right place, and she is undoubtedly making a lasting impact in the world of health and wellbeing.

My personal and professional experiences with Dr Charlton have always been nothing short of delightful. Her unwavering enthusiasm for health and wellness deserves recognition and celebration. She's not only a dedicated and knowledgeable doctor, but also a deeply family-oriented person who finds joy in sharing her success and wisdom with others. Dr Avi Charlton is a beautiful example of someone using her gifts to uplift and inspire the lives around her, and the world is better for it."

Laura Gindac,
Founder of *XQ-SLESS WELLNESS*

"In a world full of confusing diet advice and quick fixes, Dr Avi Charlton's book, 'Prescribing Lifestyle', feels like a wise friend gently guiding you back to what really works. Avi isn't just a doctor – she's someone who has faced her own struggles and learned how to make real, lasting changes. This book is full of practical, down-to-earth advice that goes beyond the usual 'just eat less and move more.'

Testimonials

What I love most is how Avi breaks down the essentials into easy-to-grasp pieces, sharing the honest stories and science without confusing jargon. If you're ready to stop feeling stuck and start feeling better in your body and life, this book is the perfect place to begin!"

**Su Zaki-Leung,
TEDx Speaker, Award-Winning Entrepreneur
and Founder of *Regretless – Low Carb Pleasure***

"It's privilege to introduce 'Prescribing Lifestyle'. This book captures the essence of Dr Avi Charlton's medical philosophy: lasting health begins not with restriction or prescriptions, but with empowerment, education, and curiosity.

I have had the honour of working alongside Avi for many years. She is a General Practitioner who brings clinical expertise, deep compassion, and relentless dedication to improving the lives of her patients. Her interest in low-carbohydrate nutrition, metabolic health, and breathwork is not theoretical – it is embodied in her practice, her teaching, and her way of life. She constantly explores innovative ways to help people take control of their health, whether through digital programs, her Prescribing Lifestyle podcast, or personalised care.

I particularly admire Avi's commitment to helping patients create meaningful, sustainable lifestyle changes that not only improve their well-being but, in many cases, allow for the safe deprescribing of medications. This is where true healing begins:

when patients no longer just manage symptoms but actually reverse the course of chronic illness.

In 'Prescribing Lifestyle', Avi generously shares her journey alongside the clinical evidence. From her transformation to the evolution of her social media presence – shifting from 'Low Carb GP' to 'Lifestyle GP' – her message has remained unwavering: that we all deserve to feel empowered in our health. Her identity and purpose have remained clear, even as her knowledge and reach have expanded.

This book is not about fads or perfection. It's about clarity amid confusion, compassion in the face of struggle, and practical, evidence-based steps towards lifelong wellbeing. Avi's voice is warm, grounded, and encouraging, feeling as though your trusted GP is right there beside you, helping you make one positive shift at a time.

This book offers a refreshing alternative if you've ever felt overwhelmed by conflicting health advice or frustrated by short-term fixes. Dr Avi Charlton reminds us that health is not something to chase – it's something we build, habit by habit, breath by breath. You are in good hands."

Dr Angela Kwong, MBBS DCH FRACGP,
Founder of *Enlighten Me*

Testimonials

"Dr Avi Charlton is a passionate doctor who is as honest as the day is long. Her dedication to her patients is evident in her relentless pursuit of knowledge and her commitment to sharing it.

Dr Avi Charlton's 'Prescribing Lifestyle' is a book that genuinely meets people where they are. It's a practical, down-to-earth guide that helps readers make sense of the confusing world of health and nutrition. Avi writes with warmth and authenticity, sharing her own journey and the stories of her patients, making it clear that lasting change isn't about quick fixes or willpower, but about understanding how our bodies work and what truly nourishes us. She walks readers through the essentials – nutrition, movement, sleep, stress management, community, and breaking free from addictive habits – offering simple steps anyone can take to feel better and stay healthier.

As a lifestyle medicine doctor and someone who cares deeply about evidence-based, patient-centred care, I highly recommend this book to anyone looking for a realistic, compassionate path to better health."

Dr Lucy Burns,
Co-Founder of *Real Life Medicine*

"Avi is the most inspiring, courageous, open-minded and level-headed human being, always bringing out the best in others. Over our 30+ years of friendship, she has been a rock to lean and rely on. She has the most amazing passion for encouraging and advocating for everyone around her to adopt long-lasting, sustainable lifestyle changes that ultimately bring good health, quality of life and happiness. Her enthusiasm never ceases to amaze me!"

**Assoc Prof Valerie Sung,
Paediatrician and Researcher**

"As a long-time personal trainer, health retreat facilitator, and behaviour change coach, I am deeply committed to supporting lasting transformation in women's health and wellbeing. I have had the privilege of working professionally and collaboratively alongside Dr Avi Charlton, most recently while co-hosting our Mansfield Keto-based intermittent fasting retreat.

Her rare blend of medical expertise, compassion, and willingness to question the status quo sets her apart. Avi doesn't just treat symptoms; she empowers people to understand what's driving them in the first place. Her approach aligns so closely with what I've witnessed time and again in my own work: that real, sustainable change only comes when we support the whole person, not with restriction or punishment, but with education, simplicity, and care.

This book is like having her in the room with you, calmly debunking myths, guiding you through the noise, and offering a clear, compassionate framework for achievable health, deeply rooted in science.

Whether you're starting or starting again, Prescribing Lifestyle is the book I wish every one of my clients had in their hands."

Julie Bristow
Coach, Retreat Facilitator and Founder of
Rejuvenate Health Retreats

"Dr Avi Charlton is a trailblazer in the world of lifestyle medicine. As a fellow medical professional, I am inspired by her courage to challenge conventional norms and her dedication to exploring the root causes of chronic disease rather than merely treating symptoms. 'Prescribing Lifestyle' is a deeply personal yet scientifically grounded guide that reflects Dr Charlton's commitment to empowering her patients with real, lasting solutions.

What sets Avi apart is her authentic voice—she speaks not only as a doctor but as someone who has walked the same journey as many of her patients. Her blend of clinical expertise, lived experience, and compassion brings both credibility and heart to her work. Through this book, she equips readers with practical tools, nutritional insights, and a deep understanding of the pillars of vibrant health.

Dr Charlton exemplifies what modern medicine should look like: integrative, evidence-informed, and patient-centred. This book is a powerful resource for anyone ready to take back control of their health—and a must-read for healthcare professionals who are ready to do the same."

Dr Olivia Ong, Pain Medicine Physician, Professional Speaker, Best-selling Author, and Founder of *The Heart Centred Method Institute*

DEDICATION

—— ◆◇◆ ——

To my patients, thank you for trusting me as your doctor. You shared your journey, health, and struggles with me and taught me how to be compassionate.

To my family and friends, thank you for your ongoing support, patience, and love.

To my supporters, podcast listeners, and every reader, may I inspire you to keep learning.

May this book be a starting point to lasting change and vibrant health.

CONTENTS

————————— ◆◇◆ —————————

FOREWORD

———————— ◆◇◆ ————————

"I find it hard to believe that Avi Charlton was ever a 'busy GP who was overweight, tired and lacking energy.' The Avi Charlton I know has boundless energy, enormous enthusiasm and is an inspiration to many. The best health practitioners are often those who have experienced their own health problems and have found a solution which starts them on a broader journey of discovery. Avi has been on that journey and the lessons she has learned; she now puts into practice guiding her patients on their own journeys of discovery.

Initially Avi's focus was on diet – reducing carbs and processed foods and focussing on real foods - and exercise, two of her six essentials for improving health and well-being. But Avi understands that there is more to health then just diet and exercise. Her other four essential elements are sleep, stress management, community support and managing addictions. Avi provides heaps of practical advice for managing all six elements.

This wonderful book takes the reader on a journey of discovery that will be life-changing for many of you. I encourage you to read it from cover to cover – there are unexpected pearls of wisdom on every page – and then go back to the sections of the book that resonate most with you. If you follow Avi's simple guidelines for a healthy life, I promise you will be considerably healthier and happier.

I am not sure where Avi found the time to write this book in between a hectic family life with two children, her busy medical practice, 'Melbourne Low Carb Clinic', her running, including parkruns and marathons, her recent interest in meditation and breathwork, her speaking schedule, and her 'Prescribing Lifestyle' podcast. I am exhausted just thinking about all that! But I am glad she did – and so will you be.

Avi Charlton is a remarkable doctor who has changed the lives of hundreds of her patients. This book deserves a broader audience and the opportunity to help so many of us on our life journey with all its challenges.

Enjoy the read."

Professor Peter Brukner OAM, MBBS, FACSEP
Professor of Sports Medicine at *La Trobe University*,
Founder of *SugarByHalf* and *Defeat Diabetes* and Author
of *A Fat Lot of Good* and *The Diabetes Plan*

INTRODUCTION

THE PRESCRIPTION YOU WERE NEVER GIVEN

———————— ◆◇◆ ————————

"The greatest medicine of all is to teach people how not to need it." (Hippocrates)

You must be so confused.

You've probably tried it all: eat less, exercise more, cut down calories, avoid all the fat, low carb, Keto, juice cleanses, intermittent fasting, exercises and still found yourself stuck, frustrated, and wondering, 'Why isn't this working?'

What if I told you that everything you've learned about diet and exercise may be missing the bigger picture? That lasting weight loss and vibrant health aren't about willpower or punishment, but about understanding how your body works, and nourishing your body.

Maybe you've asked yourself:

'Do I have to stop eating all the yummy food? Do I have to give up everything I love forever? Should I avoid fat or carbs? Is cholesterol really dangerous? Are eggs good or bad? What about snacks?'

And amidst all this conflicting advice, it's no wonder you feel overwhelmed.

I get it because I've been there, too.

As a doctor, I used to believe the same conventional advice I was trained to give. I used to tell my patients, 'Just eat less, move more.' But over time, I began to see that it doesn't work for my patients or myself.

So, I went on a journey of unlearning, relearning, and rediscovering. I explored the science behind metabolism, which means how our body works. This includes nutrition, stress, sleep, movement and even breathing, and a whole lot more.

This book is about my journey.

This book isn't going to give you all the answers so you can live happily ever after. It's about empowering you to keep learning, explore the science, and understand how it applies to your own body. You would need to try out what works best for yourself. I hope that it inspires you to embark on your own journey, one of discovery, growth, and ongoing curiosity. I don't claim to know it all. I will keep learning, and hopefully this will inspire you to do so, too.

Prescribing Lifestyle is the prescription you were never given. It's not a quick fix or a fad. It's a roadmap for long-lasting health, based on science, clinical experience, and real-life results. It's how I've helped countless patients lose weight, reduce medications, and feel more vibrant and energetic than they have in years.

I will share with you a few patients' journeys. Their stories aren't the same as yours, but they may inspire you to continue to learn. You will learn about the history, the science and how it may relate to your own health.

Let me show you a new way forward – one that is empowering, nourishing, and sustainable. One that puts you back in control of your health.

Ready? Let's begin.

The Story of a Fat Doctor

I remember back in 2017, I was a busy GP and a working mum. I was in my 40s with two young boys, aged six and nine. I was tired, juggling work, parenting, cooking, cleaning, grocery shopping, and everything that comes with running a household.

One day, a patient came in for her regular prescription. In a casual, friendly manner, she asked, 'When are you due for your third baby?'

I was floored and shocked because I wasn't pregnant. I was speechless.

I was horrified, upset, and this moment stuck with me. I couldn't believe I had become a fat doctor. I couldn't believe that I was giving health advice to my patients, but I was unable to control my own weight. I need to start looking after my own health.

Determined to take action, I joined the local gym and started going to classes three times a week.

After a few months, I did not lose a kilogram, but I did feel slightly more energetic. Frustrated and looking for a new way, my gym instructor happened to be running an eight-week body transformation challenge. I love new challenges and am always up for one, so I said, 'Yes, sign me up.'

The eight-week body transformation challenge involved gym classes as often as possible. I went three times a week, including strength training sessions and bootcamp sessions. I was also given a spreadsheet on which I had to weigh all my food on a scale. I remember putting 120 grams of protein, 20 grams of fat, and 20 grams of carbs on the scale. It was precise, meticulous, but surprisingly doable.

After eight weeks, I won the challenge by losing 4% body fat and 4kg of weight. I had also built a little bit of muscle. 4kg may not sound much to you, but I am a very petite Asian woman, only five feet tall. I noticed my belly was much slimmer, and I was ecstatic.

My boss at the time had noticed I had lost a bit of weight and asked me how. He guessed that I had 'gone Keto'. He was envious. I didn't know what Keto was and deep-dived into a new rabbit hole of research.

Keto, I learnt, stands for ketogenic. It refers to a metabolic state called ketosis, in which the body changes from burning glucose to burning fat for energy.

The more I read, the more I was intrigued and keen to continue to learn. I learnt about my body. What amazed me was that I had stopped feeling hungry. The usual 'hangry' doctor, who by mid-morning needed a snack, had enough energy to continue powering on till lunchtime. I felt satiated and didn't need a snack.

I continued gym classes three times a week, but also decided to take up running. I downloaded a free app called *Couch to 5 K* (C25K), gradually building up running more and more. It became a time when I could be with myself. I escaped the constant demands of work and motherhood and stepping outside into nature.

I am lucky enough to live near bushland. I have kangaroos living in a bush park near my house. I listened to music, looked at the kangaroos and took pictures of them, enjoyed nature, and found myself some me-time. I walked when running was too hard.

I also discovered *parkrun,* a free initiative that originated in the United Kingdom. There are many locally run parkruns that are run by volunteers. At these weekly events, I made friends who lived in my neighbourhood. I discovered a sense of support, community, and connection.

In 2019, I attended a conference organised by *Low Carb Down Under* for health professionals. It was the first time I discovered a group of doctors who had similar journeys. Many of them have journeys of weight loss, improving health, and personal transformation.

I learnt from Dr Peter Brukner, Dr Gary Fettke, Dr Paul Mason, Dr Lucy Burns, Dr Rob Szabo, and many more. These doctors learnt from their personal experiences, started incorporating them into their medical practice, and helped their patients reverse chronic diseases, come off medications and regain their lives.

And I thought, 'Why aren't we all practising this way?'

This was the turning point. I couldn't keep prescribing the same way. I had to keep learning about nutrition, lifestyle, and how to incorporate it into my general practice.

That is the beginning of my journey of *Prescribing Lifestyle*.

The Weight Loss Struggle We've All Seen

As I reflect on my journey as a GP, I realise many of my patients share a similar story. The majority of them are middle-aged women, maybe around 50. They may be juggling busy lives, including work, running a household, and other stressful events in life. Many of them are struggling with weight loss.

They may have tried numerous diets, some worked for a short period, but left them tired, with no energy, and unsustainable. They feel helpless, confused, and stuck in a cycle of weight gain. They begin to feel frustrated and unattractive to their partners, which can lead to feelings of depression and loss of self-esteem. It is a difficult, emotional journey that leaves them questioning their self-worth.

Many try diets, including *Jenny Craig*, *Weight Watchers*, calorie counting, 'eat less and move more', and even weight loss medications or injections. Some people have some success, lose a few kilograms, but find their weight creeping back on. Some have found they lose motivation, or cravings and hunger win out. Some may find messages confusing with so much information out there, and it's hard to know who and what to trust.

For example, some sources claim red meat is harmful, advocating plant-based or vegan diets. For a long time, we've been worried about eating eggs because of worries about cholesterol. Most diets advocate for calorie reduction and even starvation, leaving people with increased cravings, hunger, and feelings of deprivation. The conflicting advice leaves people overwhelmed and unsure which direction to take.

I've heard all these stories in consultations. I have gone down that track myself as well. In the following chapters, we'll dive into how we got here. We'll learn about science and how our body works. I'll try to explain hormones and how our body works in simple, easy-to-understand terms.

The Current Health Crisis No One Talks About

It breaks my heart to see the obesity rate climbing higher and higher. According to the *World Health Organisation* (WHO), obesity rates have doubled from 7% in 1990 to 16% in 2022.[1] The global obesity rate has risen significantly across all age groups. In men, the obesity rate rose from 4.8% to 14%. In women, obesity rates increased from 8.8% to 18.5%.[2] In Australia, the statistics are even more alarming, with two-thirds (66%) of adults classified as overweight or obese.[3]

Globally, over 1 billion people are living with obesity.[4]

And it's not just adults. Child and adolescent obesity rates quadrupled globally from 2% in 1990 to 8% in 2022.[5] These statistics hit home as both a GP and a mother. Over the 20 years of being a GP, I have seen more and more overweight children coming through the doors. I also witness that my children's friends are increasingly overweight. Some parents bring their kids in, worried and unsure of how to manage their child's weight in a world of mixed messages and unhealthy habits. It's heartbreaking. It's a sign that we need a new approach.

Diabetes rates also soared. In 1990, 7% of the population had type 2 diabetes. This has risen to 14% in 2022.[6]

Chronic diseases that aren't caused by infections, like heart disease, diabetes, cancer, Alzheimer's disease, arthritis, and mental health conditions, have all increased across the board. In 2023, 60% of all Australians are living with at least one chronic condition. This figure used to be 42% in 2007. [7]

And what conditions are growing the fastest? Mental health and behavioural disorders. Arthritis, back pains, asthma, Chronic Obstructive Airways Disease (COAD) and diabetes are all increasing in prevalence. Heart disease is still the leading cause of death, but dementia is expected to overtake it in the coming years.

The link between these conditions is that most of them can be influenced by our lifestyle, i.e. diet, movement, stress, sleep, and environment. Many factors are at play, including genetics, but modifying our lifestyle can often mitigate what we inherit. I love the saying, 'Genetics load the gun, but lifestyle pulls the trigger.'

In my 20 years as a GP, I've seen firsthand that obesity, diabetes, and many chronic conditions are not just creeping up; they are exploding.

In 2020 and 2021, we had a totally different illness. We endured the COVID-19 pandemic. I live in Melbourne, which became known as the most locked-down city globally. We experienced six lockdowns between March 2020 and October 2021, totalling 262 days.[8] The toll on mental and physical health was immense.

But while we were all worried about the effects and deaths of COVID-19 and urging vaccinations, we have not realised that diabetes quietly killed more people.

In 2022, diabetes was linked to approximately 21,900 deaths in Australia, about 11% of all deaths that year.[9] In contrast, COVID-19 was linked to 9,859 deaths, or 5.2% of total deaths.[10]

Our Victorian Premier appeared on television almost daily, urging the population to stay indoors and get vaccinated. However, similar health advice does not encourage the population to eat healthy, exercise, and maintain a healthy lifestyle.

People with diabetes often face a range of serious complications, including vision loss, amputations, kidney disease, heart disease, slow wound healing, diabetic feet, and the list goes on. It's not just the increased risk of early death; it has a significant impact on quality of life and long-term health span.

We are significantly losing years in health span. In Australia, the current life expectancy is around 84 years.[11] However, our current health-adjusted life expectancy, i.e. health span, is about 72 years.[12] This means on average; people are living 12 years in poor health.

It is time we start paying more attention to the current health crisis that's been building and worsening. It's not just about numbers. It's about real lives, families, children, and real suffering. It's time we look into advocating and prescribing a lifestyle so people can be empowered to take charge of their health.

My Journey in Learning About Lifestyle Medicine

I graduated from the *University of Melbourne* medical school in 2000 after completing six years of training. In medical school, I was taught how to recognise patients with heart attacks, infections, and emergencies and how to deal with them. It didn't occur to me that little attention was given to preventive care.

After graduating from medical school, I worked as a junior doctor at *Box Hill Hospital* for three years. I gained experience in various departments, including medical wards, surgical wards, and the emergency department, and I even delivered babies in the middle of the night. My journey also took me to regional hospitals, where I cared for Australia's Aboriginal community.

I remember during those years of hospital work, I witnessed firsthand devastating complications of many chronic conditions, such as diabetes. I worked in the operating theatre helping surgeons with amputating toes or feet of diabetic patients with blocked arteries. I saw chronic diabetic foot ulcers that wouldn't heal. I also see diabetic patients with eye disease going blind. But I didn't know these conditions were preventable.

I went into General Practice because I want to help people, cure illnesses, and make a difference. I want to have a broad knowledge base of a person's health rather than specialising in one body part. For the first 15 years of my practice, I followed prescribing guidelines. Patients with high blood pressure were given antihypertensives, and I prescribed antidepressants for those who were depressed. I did not know there was another way. I treated countless patients with infections, mental health issues, diabetes, cancer, and weight loss struggles.

But it wasn't until 2019, when I attended the *Low Carb Down Under* conference for doctors, that I reflected on my practice. For nearly two decades, I had been treating symptoms and prescribing medications for symptoms without looking into the root cause of the illnesses I was managing. The conference sparked my shift in thinking and opened my eyes to the importance of addressing nutrition and lifestyle factors in my patients' health.

Then, I started to explore nutrition and recognise how important our food is to our health. I learnt the importance of eating nutrient-dense foods and understood how our hormones work to regulate hunger, satiety, and weight regulation. I realised our body can only tolerate a certain amount of glucose in the bloodstream before our hormones go awry. I realised the calories in and calories out model doesn't work. There is an intricate relationship between our food and health, which often contributes to diseases and illnesses.

As I dive deeper into my research, I experiment with my nutrition and health. I adopted a whole-food approach to my diet. I started to see an improvement in my energy levels and overall well-being. I did not just lose 4kg, but I also had more energy and mental clarity and was less hungry. I began to prescribe more nutritious, low-carbohydrate diets for my patients, especially those with less carbohydrate tolerance. These are patients who want to lose weight and those with diabetes. The outcomes were remarkable. Patients started losing weight, feeling less hungry, experiencing less bloating and improved in their blood test metabolic markers. Hypertension improved, and patients managed to escape the prescription pad of medications.

I began learning the practice of de-prescribing – the careful and supervised reduction of medications that are no longer needed. In medical school, we were taught how to prescribe medications for chronic diseases. Nobody taught us how to take medications away. As I started focusing on nutrition, I saw remarkable changes in my patients.

Often, patients realise they may not need as many medications as they used to, and I began to de-prescribe. Many diabetic and hypertensive medications were able to be stopped. De-prescribing has become one of the most rewarding parts of my work. I helped patients to be empowered not just to manage their disease, but to heal and regain independence from their long-term medications.

This approach to prescribing nutrition has made my work more rewarding than ever. I began seeing patients return with positive results. Some lost weight and managed to keep it off. I had a mum who struggled to fall pregnant for nine years, got her period back and conceived naturally. Other patients with aches and pains controlled their pain and inflammation by eating better.

Eager to continue learning, I enrolled in courses with *Nutrition Network*, a company from South Africa that provides online learning. I read books like *The Big Fat Lie* by Nina Teicholz, which discusses the history of our diet, and *Why We Get Sick* by Ben Bikman, which explains how hormones work in our body. All this deepened my understanding of nutrition, metabolic health, and how our bodies work. I also pursued additional courses with the *Australasian College of Environmental Medicine* (ACNEM), where I learnt to integrate nutrition and environmental medicine into my practice, further expanding my knowledge and approach to patient care.

This journey of discovery not only transformed my approach to medicine but also reignited my passion for helping patients through lifestyle changes. Not only did I learn about nutrition, but I also delved into other pillars of lifestyle, including incorporating sleep and stress management.

Taking Control of My Health: A Personal Journey

As I committed to a low-carb way of eating, I made several changes, including focusing more on protein, including meat, eggs, chicken, and fish. I mostly eat above-ground vegetables, as the below-ground vegetables are often more starchy. I also stopped eating bread, which has been a staple in my diet. I realised that all carbohydrates are basically glucose molecules linked together.

Being Chinese, rice has always been a staple. I grew up eating rice and noodles with every meal. It is an integral part of my culture and upbringing. However, knowing that rice can lead to glucose spikes, I decided to remove it from my diet. It wasn't easy, but it was a necessary step in managing my health.

Understanding how the foods impact my body changed the way I approached eating. I paid attention to nourishment and what truly supports my health. I try not to focus on deprivation, but instead on making choices that are right for me and help me feel my best. I do my best, and if I slip up, I don't beat myself up. If I enjoy a cake at a birthday party and enjoy the party, I don't beat myself up. What matters most is what I put in my body most of the time.

In addition to these dietary changes, I also focused on other aspects of my lifestyle. I continued to enjoy strength training, attending the gym twice a week. I started my running journey with the *C25K* app, then 5km parkrun, and progressed to running half marathons. Eventually, I completed two full marathons, 42km each. The *Oxfam* challenge, walking 100km up massive mountains, was a real challenge. I had setbacks, including a couple of fractures of my foot and shin splints, but ultimately, these have built my strength and resilience.

Alongside physical exercises, I began exploring meditation and mindfulness techniques. In 2023, I discovered breathwork and functional breathing techniques. This has been a game changer in managing my stress and busy lifestyle. I went on to become a breathwork facilitator, which helped me prescribe helpful breathing techniques to patients for not only stress and anxiety but also for helping their sleep, asthma, and respiratory conditions.

How I Became an Entrepreneur

As a regular GP, working in a bulk billing clinic, it was never an issue trying to find patients. I had a plethora of infections, immunisations, mental illnesses, and inflammatory conditions that filled my appointment book.

As I learnt about nutrition, I decided to list my name under the *Low Carb Down Under* website's doctors' list. Many found me from all over Melbourne and across Australia. Some travelled from the other side of the city to consult a doctor who would discuss nutrition. Many patients have already adopted a low-carb lifestyle and need help with their blood tests. Some didn't feel supported by their usual GP and came to see me. Some felt they weren't listened to. Many felt their doctor just wanted to put them on medication.

I started sharing my journey on social media as 'Dr Charlton Low Carb GP.' I would share some talks, what I cook with my family, and even my running adventures. As I learnt more about other lifestyle pillars, I renamed my handle 'Dr Charlton's Lifestyle GP.' I connected with many like-minded health coaches and nutritionists and found a community and friendship. I had also started being invited to talk about my journey and the science behind this lifestyle.

In August 2022, I woke up one Sunday morning and told my husband, 'I want to set up my own low-carb clinic,' and started brainstorming with him and a few friends. I approached the principal of my clinic, whom I had worked for over 15 years. He was happy to rent out a room for me to start this journey. This became the start of *Melbourne Low Carb Clinic*.

I set out on a mission to continue learning. This included all aspects of lifestyle, including exercise, stress management, sleep, the power of community support, and managing addictions.

I am also on a mission to spread the message. I talk about it to patients who come to the low-carb clinic and those who come in for other medical conditions. I aspire to become a speaker and advocate for lifestyle medicine, focusing on empowering individuals to optimise their lives.

I am not anti-medication – far from it. I believe in a balanced, integrated approach where lifestyle interventions work alongside medications to support weight loss, improve energy, reverse chronic conditions, and promote long-term health and longevity. This approach puts patients back in the driver's seat of their health journey, encouraging them to take ownership, keep learning and become active participants rather than passive recipients of care.

The Six Pillars of Lifestyle Medicine: Essential Elements for Improving Health and Well-Being

Nutrition: We'll explore the myths and misconceptions that dominate the world of nutrition. Together, we'll debunk the confusion that has fuelled the diet wars and unravel how we arrived at the current state of dietary guidelines.

Exercise or Movement: It's time to rethink exercise. Rather than focusing on working out to lose weight, we'll discuss how building strength through muscle development is key to overall health and longevity.

Sleep: Prioritising sleep is essential for health. We'll delve into the importance of circadian rhythms, understanding how our bodies function under the master clock, and why aligning with natural sleep cycles is crucial for our well-being.

Stress Management: Stress is the root cause of many diseases. We'll examine how past traumas and experiences shape our ability to manage stress and explore practical strategies for transforming how we respond to the stressors in our lives.

Community Support: Support from family, friends, and our communities is just as vital as the other pillars. We'll examine the importance of building a supportive tribe and how these relationships play a critical role in our health and happiness.

Managing Addictions: Addiction isn't just about substances like alcohol or cigarettes – it can also involve food or even dopamine-driven habits, such as screen and social media addiction. We'll discuss these less-talked-about forms of addiction and how they impact our mental and physical health.

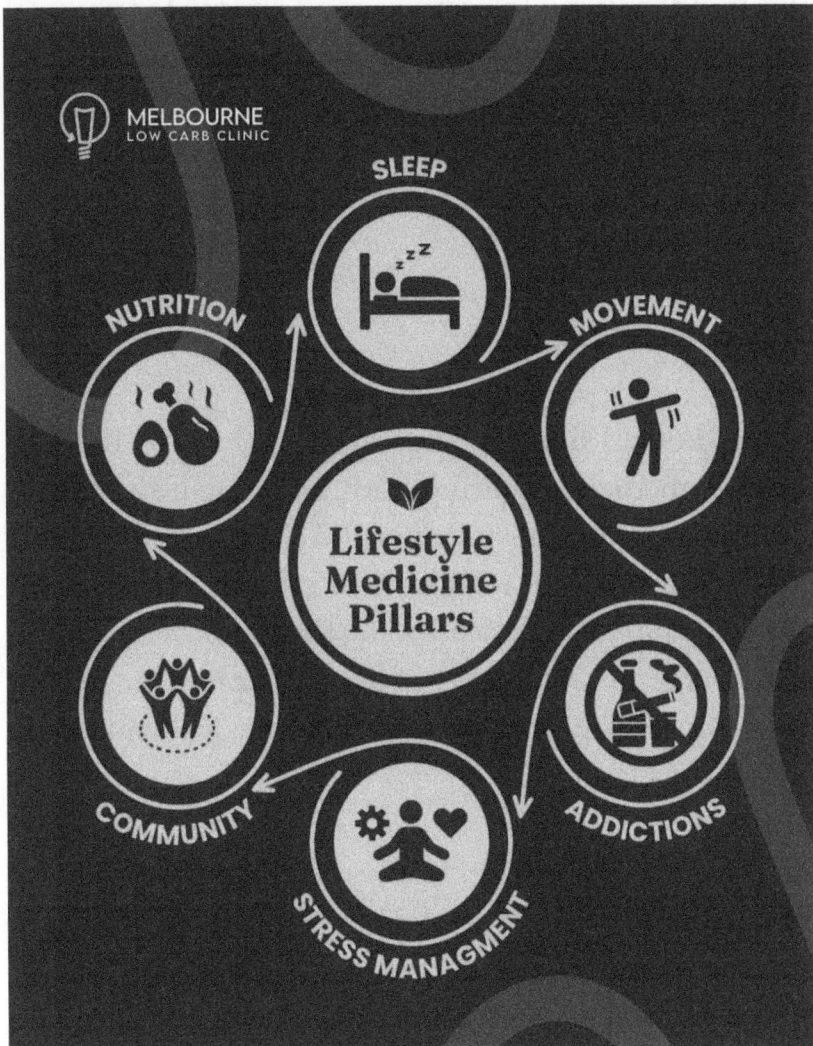

The six pillars of lifestyle medicine help each other. They are intertwined and deeply connected and work synergistically to support optimum health, prevent, and even reverse chronic diseases. Working on one pillar helps the other five.

For example, eating healthy nutrition fuels your body and mind, helping to provide good energy for physical activity. This also supports sleep quality, which in turn reduces stress. With a better-fuelled body, we like to connect with our community and avoid influences from addictive substances.

How to Use This Book

In this book, I'll guide you through the six pillars of lifestyle medicine, sharing both scientific insights and real-life experiences – my own and those of my patients. For each pillar, you'll learn how simple but powerful lifestyle changes can lead to lasting improvements in health, energy, and quality of life. I'll explain the science clearly and easily so you understand not just what to do but why it works.

At the end of each section, you'll find a practical 'prescription' – a set of actionable steps to help you begin making positive changes. Some may be minor tweaks; others might feel like bigger shifts. You don't have to do everything at once. Progression, not perfection, is the goal. This is your journey, and it's meant to be sustainable. I will also give you some resources, such as books or people you can research to learn more about the topic further.

That said, the benefit you get from this book depends on your mindset. Those who are open-minded and willing to unlearn old habits and relearn new ones will likely see the most success. If you've been thinking, 'I've tried it all,' this approach might not work for you unless you're ready to challenge those beliefs. If you're the type of person who enjoys exploring different ideas and is willing to dive into new rabbit holes, this book will empower you to experiment, review, and try different approaches until you find what works for you.

Remember, everyone is different. You are your own coach. It's essential to explore your own body, pay attention to what it's telling you, and discover the changes that make the most difference for your unique needs. I'm here to guide you, but ultimately, you'll be the one in control of your health journey.

It's also important to note that if you have chronic conditions, especially if you are taking medications, please consult with your doctor before making any significant changes to your diet or lifestyle. Your medications may need to be adjusted. For example, people with diabetes who are on insulin or oral medications may need their doses reduced as they adopt a low-carb diet, as their blood glucose may drop too low. Likewise, those on medication for high blood pressure may need dose adjustments as their diet and health improve. Always consult your doctor to ensure these changes are made safely.

Supporting patients through this process – witnessing their transformation as they adopt lifestyle changes and often reduce or even eliminate medications – has been one of the most fulfilling parts of my work as a doctor. I hope this book inspires and equips you to take meaningful steps toward lasting health.

Your First Prescription

- Be curious.
- Have an open mind. You might need to unlearn to relearn.
- Start the journey by downloading my free eBook, *How To Start Low Carb*. https://mlcclinic.com.au/free-resources/

DISCLAIMER

— ◆◇◆ —

This book shares real-life stories of how individuals, patients and friends have improved their health through lifestyle changes. These case studies are included to educate, inspire, and encourage readers to explore how nutrition, movement, stress management, and other lifestyle factors can influence well-being.

All case studies have been de-identified to protect confidentiality, and I have followed the *Australian Health Practitioner Regulation Agency (AHPRA)* guidelines for sharing patient information.

Please note that the successes described in these stories are individual experiences and may not apply to everyone. If you have a medical condition or take medications, you should always consult your own doctor or a qualified health professional before making changes to your health routine.

The information in this book is for general educational purposes only and is not intended to be a substitute for personalised medical advice, diagnosis, or treatment.

PART 1

Just Eat Real Food

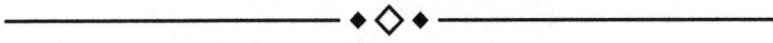

—————◆◇◆—————

CHAPTER 1

NUTRITION: FUELLING YOUR BODY FOR HEALTH AND WEIGHT LOSS

◆◇◆

*"Food is the most powerful tool we have
to heal and transform our health."*
(Mark Hyman)

Sarah was 49 when she came to see me. She wanted to lose weight, regain her energy, get back on her bike, and be active again. At that time, she was 115kg with a BMI of 51, falling into the 'morbidly obese' category. In addition, she also suffered from asthma and ongoing back and leg pain from a car accident many years earlier.

Her usual breakfast was bacon and eggs with toast or a wrap, and dinner was often whatever was available, typically pasta or rice with some form of protein. As a personal carer, she was always on the move, driving between clients, which made consistent meal choices challenging. She believed she was eating healthy.

Through a few initial consultations, we focused on cutting back on foods that weren't supporting her weight loss goals. She began prioritising high-quality protein and above-ground vegetables. When on the road, she made simple but effective swaps – like choosing sashimi from a food court, ordering a bun-less burger from a fast food place, or picking up roast chicken or souvlaki meat without the wrap from the supermarket.

Driven and committed, Sarah started coming in every two weeks for coaching and accountability. Over the first year, she lost around 10kg. In the following year, her weight stabilised with a minor regain of 2kg-3kg, settling at a BMI of around 41 – a significant improvement from where she began.

Beyond the number on the scale, her health noticeably improved. She experienced fewer asthma attacks, and her chronic pain became more manageable. I also observed improvements in her speech and mental clarity – something she noticed, too.

While sometimes she feels she was off track, she's learned not to be discouraged by them. She would try to learn from the experience and get back on track. She knows what works for her body and what she needs to do. Most importantly, she continues to move forward and progress over perfection.

In fact, I have many stories of patients just like Sarah. Often, they're surprised no one ever explained that carbohydrates act like sugar in the body. They're also shocked that their previous doctors prescribed medications for diabetes without teaching them how to eat in a way that supports their health.

I've worked with numerous patients who have been able to reduce or even stop their diabetes and blood pressure medications. Many find their way to me after discovering this lifestyle on their own and are simply looking for a doctor who will support them on their journey.

CHAPTER 2

HOW DID WE GET HERE? THE HISTORY AND BATTLES OF THE DIET WARS

———————— ◆◇◆ ————————

Y ou may be very confused about what to eat. You are not alone. The messages are very confusing. One day, fat is the villain. The next day, it's sugar and carbs. There have been many mixed messages throughout the years. Some messages say glucose is essential for exercise and brain function. Fat has been the demon for many years, as we worry about increasing our body fat from eating fat. We are confused about saturated fat vs polyunsaturated fats. We question food labels, organic vs non-organic.

The truth is the world of nutrition has a long history of diet wars. The wars between low-fat, low-carb, and high-protein diets are leaving us more and more confused.

But how did we get here? In this chapter, I'll take you on a brief journey through the history of how we got into such a confused state.

But first of all, let's take you back millions of years, when our ancestors were hunter-gatherers. Imagine what they would eat. They would hunt animals and feast when they had gathered meat. When meat wasn't available, they would turn to fruit and vegetables to sustain themselves.

Fast-forward many generations, and our grandparents ate simple, wholesome meals, such as meat and vegetables. In the colder months, some cultures rely on cured meats and preserved vegetables.

So, how did we go from this natural eating method to today's confusing mess? In this chapter, I will explain the history of how we got here.

The Surprising Origins of Our Dietary Guidelines

The way we eat today didn't come about purely through science – it's the result of a complex mix of religious beliefs, influential personalities, political decisions, and well-meaning but flawed public health policies.

Much of this has been thoroughly researched and documented by Belinda Fettke[13], whose work you can explore further on *YouTube* and online. She's spent years uncovering how our dietary guidelines were shaped, and I encourage you to look into her work if this topic sparks your curiosity. For now, let me give you a brief overview.

Religious Roots: Ellen G. White and the Seventh-Day Adventist Influence

In the late 1800s, Ellen G. White, a woman who claimed to be a prophet, co-founded the *Seventh-Day Adventist Church*.[14] She believed that meat consumption stimulated impure thoughts and that vegetarianism was the path to spiritual purity. These beliefs became central to the Adventist health message – a message that still strongly influences their dietary recommendations today.

One of her devoted followers was Dr John Harvey Kellogg, a physician and staunch Adventist who ran the famous *Battle Creek Sanitarium*. He was a vocal advocate for vegetarianism, hydrotherapy, and abstinence – not just from alcohol and tobacco, but also sex. To promote a bland, meatless diet that suppressed libido, he invented *Cornflakes*, marking the birth of the breakfast cereal industry.

These two important figures laid the foundations of the *Seventh-Day Adventist Church*. Their teachings were the precursors of plant-based nutrition. They also contributed to the training of health professionals, including dieticians, nurses, and physicians.

The Fat vs Sugar Debate: Yudkin vs Keys

Fast forward to the mid-20th century. Heart disease had become a leading cause of death, and scientists were racing to uncover why seemingly 'healthy' men were dying of heart attacks in their 40s and 50s.

Two competing theories emerged:

- Professor John Yudkin, a British physiologist, blamed sugar. In his book *Pure, White and Deadly*[15], he warned that hidden sugars in breakfast cereals, processed foods, and soft drinks were fuelling obesity, diabetes, and heart disease.
- On the other side was Ancel Keys, an American scientist with charisma, political clout, and a strong belief that saturated fat was the villain. His Seven Countries study[16] suggested a link between saturated fat and heart disease – but critics have since noted he selectively included data that supported his theory and excluded countries that didn't.

Despite the debate, Keys' theory won out. His message was simpler, easier to package, and aligned with public health efforts to reduce heart disease. By 1977, the first U.S. Dietary Guidelines were released[17], urging the public to reduce fat, particularly saturated fat, and replace it with grains and carbohydrates. Australia and other nations soon followed suit.

Enter: The Processed Food Industry

This shift gave rise to a powerful new player – Big Food.

As people were told to avoid fat, food companies filled the gap with low-fat products that were instead loaded with added sugars, refined carbohydrates, and seed oils to maintain taste and texture. Yogurts, cereals, muesli bars, snack packs – even cookies – were now marketed as 'healthy' simply because they were low in fat.

But the results were disastrous. Over the following decades, obesity, type 2 diabetes, and metabolic syndrome surged. Despite eating less fat, we were becoming sicker and more overweight than ever before.

Yudkin's warnings about sugar and processed foods were ignored for years, only to be rediscovered decades later, as the evidence began to shift.

Why the Dietary Guidelines Don't Work for Most People

The official dietary guidelines were created with good intentions: to reduce chronic disease and promote public health. But here's the problem – these guidelines were designed for metabolically healthy individuals, who are people with normal weight, normal blood sugar, healthy blood pressure, and no signs of insulin resistance.

According to the *National Health and Medical Research Council* (NHMRC), the Australian Dietary Guidelines apply to all healthy Australians.[18] They do not apply to those who need special dietary advice for a medical condition.

But today, over half of adults are metabolically unhealthy. Many are already living with weight issues, high blood sugar, fatty liver, pre-diabetes, type 2 diabetes, or heart disease. For these people, following the standard low-fat, high-carb guidelines may actually be doing more harm than good.

And here's the kicker – we *have* followed the guidelines.

As a society, we're eating less red meat[19], less saturated fat than we did 50 years ago. We've cut back on protein and shifted towards more cereals, grains, low-fat dairy, seed oils, and processed snacks – just like the guidelines told us to. Yet what's happened?

- Obesity has skyrocketed
- Type 2 diabetes is on the rise
- Rates of cancer and metabolic syndrome are increasing

Clearly, something isn't working.

So, why haven't the guidelines changed?

There are many reasons for this, including vested interests, industry influence, and professional reputation. Those involved in writing the dietary guidelines have relationships with big food, beverage, and pharmaceutical companies. These companies are also responsible for sponsoring research and influencing policy. With these big companies' at stake, many influences stop the changes to the dietary guidelines.

Many professionals have been promoting low-fat, high-carb diets for decades. Admitting they are wrong could damage their credibility. Many professionals are set in their ways and would not unlearn and relearn new ways.

The standard advice may work for a small group of metabolically healthy individuals. But it fails the majority.

In fact, it may be actively contributing to the rise in chronic disease.

It's time to rethink our approach to nutrition. We need to focus on real food. This means prioritising protein and nutrient-dense whole foods, reducing processed foods and sugars.

Everyone is different, and there's no one-size-fits-all diet. However, most people, especially those with carbohydrate intolerance, should not follow the standard dietary guidelines.

So, what should we do instead? What does science say?

CHAPTER 3

UNDERSTANDING SCIENCE: WHAT'S BEHIND YOUR PLATE

——————— ◆◇◆ ———————

To understand nutrition, we must first understand its basic building blocks – the three macronutrients: **protein, fat,** and **carbohydrates**. Each of these macronutrients plays an important role in the function of your body, providing energy and supporting overall health.

Know Your Macros: The Foundations of Nutrition

Protein is made up of amino acids. These are building blocks of life, including muscles, bones, tissues, and organs. Protein is also essential for hormones and enzymes. There are **essential amino acids** that your body cannot produce, and you must obtain them from certain foods. The ideal source of amino acids comes from animal food, which provides all the essential amino acids. These include meat, eggs, chicken, and fish.

You can also get protein from plant foods like legumes, nuts, seeds, and grains. However, most plant proteins are **incomplete**, meaning they lack one or more essential amino acids. To meet your requirement for the complete profile of amino acids, you must eat a variety of protein in large quantities. The bioavailability of plant proteins is often much lower than that of animal proteins.

Protein is also very satiating, helping you feel full and satisfied, which can help with cravings and weight management.

Fat has been demonised for decades, with people fearing that eating fat will make one fat. As discussed in the chapter before, with his charismatic and convincing personality, Ancel Keys has successfully instilled the idea that eating fat will increase cholesterol. This eventually led to the dietary guidelines promoting a low-fat diet.

We now know that fat is not the enemy. In fact, fat is essential for life. It is necessary for energy, brain function, hormonal production, and cell structure. We also need fats to absorb fat-soluble vitamins (A, D, E and K). 60%

of our brain is made of fat. Omega-3 fatty acids are especially essential for brain health. These fatty acids also have anti-inflammatory effects and help regulate mood and cognitive function. Natural sources of healthy fat include avocado, nuts, seeds, dairy, olive oil, and fat found naturally in meat.

For a few decades, saturated fat has been demonised as increasing the risk of cardiovascular disease. However, in 2020, the *Journal of the American College of Cardiology* refuted this idea and published a paper stating that the current evidence does not support limiting saturated fat to reduce the risk of cardiovascular disease.[20]

It is important to note that we should avoid seed oils high in Omega-6 fatty acids. These foods include vegetable, canola, sunflower, rice bran, safflower, and margarine. These types of fats are highly processed and may promote inflammation, and some studies suggest they could increase the risk of cancer.[21] They are sold widely in supermarkets, found in processed and packaged foods, and used in restaurants to deep fry foods.

Carbohydrates are the body's quickest fuel and source of energy. When you eat carbohydrates, your body breaks them down to glucose. If you need energy, these glucose molecules will be used. However, if it is in excess, it will be stored away as fat.

When you eat carbohydrate-rich foods like bread, pasta, rice, and cereals, these are broken down into individual glucose molecules. Some may think foods like sweet potatoes, brown rice and wholemeal bread are healthy options. But they are simply slower-digesting carbohydrates that release glucose more gradually into your bloodstream.

It is important to note that carbohydrates aren't essential in the same way as proteins and fats are. While carbs give you quick energy, our bodies can also use fat as energy. We can also convert protein into glucose. This process is called gluconeogenesis. This means we can use carbs as fuel, but we don't have to. Our body functions perfectly fine without carbs. If you teach your body to burn fat and glucose, your body can become metabolically flexible, just like a hybrid vehicle that can use petrol and electric power.

Each of these macronutrients plays a role in our health, metabolism, energy use, and fat storage. But how much and in what balance we should eat depends on your individual needs and metabolic health

Too Much Sugar, Too Much Insulin, Too Much Fat

Let's discuss what happens when we eat food. Each time we eat, our body makes insulin to transport glucose to the cells to produce energy or store it as fat. Carbs raise blood glucose and subsequently insulin the most. Protein and fat will also cause the insulin to respond, but not as much as carbs.

The key is that our body can only hold 4 grams of glucose at any one time, roughly one teaspoon. This is the limit. Excess glucose is either used or stored. If you aren't burning active and burning the glucose off, the glucose is converted to fat.

To give you an idea of how much glucose is in foods:

- A can of *Coke* contains 10 teaspoons of glucose
- A bowl of *Cornflakes* contains around 8 teaspoons of glucose
- A banana contains roughly 6 teaspoons of glucose
- A single slice of white bread contains around 4 teaspoons of glucose
- A glass of apple juice contains approximately 7 teaspoons
- A bowl of rice contains nearly 10 teaspoons of glucose

Insulin is the hormone produced each time you eat. It's like a key that allows glucose to enter cells. Once inside the cell, glucose is either used immediately for energy or stored as fat for future use. Insulin ensures our blood glucose stays stable rather than allowing it to go dangerously high. If blood glucose is too high, the blood becomes sticky and inflammatory, which is what happens in diabetics when insulin fails to bring down blood glucose.

Now the problem is that insulin is working overtime when we constantly flood our bodies with glucose from carbs. Our body keeps producing more insulin to combat this. Over time, this can lead to insulin resistance – a condition where the body becomes less responsive to insulin. The insulin that is produced is no longer active. It's like the key doesn't fit into the lock anymore. Imagine a child constantly nagging his mother. Eventually, the mother becomes less responsive, even though she hears the child.

There are usually no symptoms of **insulin resistance**. Here are a few warning signs that things aren't working as well as they should. These signs include:

- **Weight gain,** particularly around the belly
- **Persistent fatigue and hunger,** even after eating
- **Skin tags,** small growths of skin typically found around the neck or armpits
- **Dark skin patches** (known as acanthosis nigricans) around the neck, elbows, or knees
- **High blood pressure**
- **Abnormal cholesterol profile** – high triglycerides and low HDL (the 'good' cholesterol)
- **Elevated fasting glucose levels** – the amount of sugar in your blood after a fast

- **Fatty liver**, which occurs when excess fat builds up in liver cells, can lead to liver disease

Insulin resistance also means the mitochondria aren't functioning correctly. Mitochondria are the powerhouses of our cells. When these mitochondria aren't functioning correctly, our cells are less efficient at using glucose and fats to produce energy. This causes the body to have a harder time functioning and producing energy.

The good news is that insulin resistance is reversible. You can improve insulin sensitivity and mitochondrial function by making the right changes in diet, lifestyle, and exercise.

Why 'Calories In, Calories Out' Doesn't Work

For years, many believe that to lose weight, we should 'eat less, and move more,' i.e., calories in, calories out. It sounds logical, except it's not as simple as that.

This theory is based on the idea that our bodies function like machines. Calories measure how much energy is produced when certain foods are put into a bomb calorimeter – the device scientists used in the early 1900s to measure energy released when they burned food. However, your body is not a bomb calorimeter.

Our body is much more complex than a machine. We have hormones. Our gut consists of many microbes that also use and produce energy. We aren't a mathematical equation.

Let's compare two foods that contain the same number of calories. A 120-gram piece of salmon contains 240 calories, and 240 calories is about one and a half cans of soft drink. They are equal in calories. However, our bodies respond to them in completely different ways. Salmon contains high-quality protein, essential Omega-3 fatty acids, and important micronutrients, such as Vitamin D, B12, B6, B3, and selenium.

Soft drinks, on the other hand, contain sugar and water. They are empty calories with no nutritional benefit. They cause a massive, rapid glucose spike and raise insulin, which works overtime to promote fat storage. Having high glucose and high insulin also increases inflammation.

Nutrient-dense foods nourish the body and keep you satiated. These foods include whole foods such as eggs, fish, meat, pork, seafood, chicken, avocado, nuts, dairy, mushrooms, and vegetables.

Conversely, foods full of empty calories include sugar, soft drinks, white flour, cakes, desserts, and processed foods. These produce energy but also trigger overeating and insulin and glucose spikes.

So, the next time someone tells you it's all about the calories, remember that it's not just about the calories; it's also how your body handles these calories.

The Hidden Danger of Constant Grazing: Why Timing Your Meals Matters

What you eat is essential, but when you eat is just as important. Every time you consume foods or drinks – whether a meal, a snack, or even milk in your coffee – your body produces insulin, the hormone responsible for letting glucose into cells.

Many people constantly graze throughout the day. They may not know that the mid-morning cafe latte with milk in the coffee or the muesli bar snack is also causing their insulin to work. Some people constantly sip sugary drinks or reach out for lollies or snacks.

Frequent insulin spikes signal your body to convert glucose into fat, making it harder to lose weight and easier to gain fat.

The world we live in is one of food abundance. We have been told that regular snacking improves metabolism. This well-meaning advice is not accurate. Constant snacking and eating contribute to insulin resistance and fuel the obesity epidemic, increasing the risk of type 2 diabetes. The more frequently you eat, the more often your body releases insulin, leading, over time, to metabolic dysfunction.

What's Really in Your Pantry? The Truth About Processed Foods

To truly continue to understand the obesity and diabetes epidemic, we must also look at the role processed foods play in it. In our fast-paced world, processed foods have become our go-to for convenience. We're conditioned to snack constantly, with kids eating sugary breakfast cereals, mid-morning 'brain food,' chips, biscuits, flavoured milk and more to 'maintain energy.'

But here's the problem: processed foods contain a toxic mix of carbohydrates, trans fats, sugar, fructose, preservatives, flavour enhancers, and artificial colourings – all of which offer little to no nutritional value.

Processed foods companies hire food technologists who work on designing foods that optimise the bliss point. When you start eating these foods, for example, *Doritos* or *Tim Tams*. Once you start, you can't stop eating at one, two or even three chips. Most people cannot control their eating until they have consumed the whole packet.

Food chemists have designed these products to be addictive, which leads to overeating and poor food choices. Not only do they wreak havoc on your gut microbiome, but they also trigger insulin responses, leading to inflammation, insulin resistance, metabolic syndrome, and eventually diabetes.

In the next chapter, I will discuss using a simple framework to plan each meal and consider ways to nourish rather than deprive. I will also discuss how your body works with hormones. We need to optimise our mitochondria and help them function at their best.

CHAPTER 4

METABOLIC MAKEOVER: FIX YOUR BLOOD SUGAR, FIX YOUR HEALTH

◆◇◆

If you want to improve your health, you must start stabilising your blood sugar. If your blood sugar fluctuates like a rollercoaster, you will feel it: fatigue, mood swings, hunger, anxiety and eventually, metabolic disease. The good news is that we can feed our bodies in a way that will help stabilise our blood sugar. I will show you a simple framework for planning your meals.

Let's keep it simple. Here's how to eat for blood sugar stability and metabolic health:

1. Prioritise Protein

When planning your meal, first consider what protein you'd like. Proteins are the building blocks for our bones, muscles, hormones, and all bodily functions. They are also the most satiating macronutrient. Protein will help you steady your blood sugar, boost your energy and mood, and keep cravings away.

For breakfast, eggs are the most straightforward and versatile choice. You can scramble, poach, fry, boil, or turn into a frittata or omelette. You can also add extras that will go with your eggs, such as mushrooms, spinach, tomatoes, avocados, cheese, chilli, bacon, sausages, or even leftover roast meat. Don't worry about the cholesterol myth.

Research has shown that dietary cholesterol does not significantly raise blood cholesterol for most people.[22] Triglycerides are what we should be looking at, with risks of cardiovascular disease.[23] At the end of the book, I will summarise what blood tests to concentrate on to look at metabolic health. In fact, eggs can help raise HDL – the 'good' cholesterol. They will improve the metabolic profile of your cholesterol profile.

If eggs aren't your thing, plenty of protein-rich, low-carb breakfast options exist – chia puddings you can make many ahead of time. Grain-free 'no oats' porridge recipes can be found. There's even a pre-made version by *Simply Swaps Food*, a local business based in the Mornington Peninsula if you're in Melbourne. Having animal proteins for breakfast, such as sausages, chicken, and beef, is unusual. That's just cultural conditioning. There is no rule that we can't have dinner food for breakfast. It's certainly much better than having cereal, which will spike your blood sugar high and drop it low as you burn off the energy quickly.

If you aren't hungry in the morning, skipping breakfast is okay. Fasting is incredibly beneficial to prevent your body from having an insulin spike. This also gives your digestive system a break. You can even have extra time to yourself by not cooking and eating breakfast. You can go outside and soak up the morning sun, or do mindfulness or breathwork to begin the day.

For lunch, I often have leftover meals from the night before. I like to cook extra protein, such as an extra steak, so I can take it to work. I have learnt to cook bacon and eggs in the microwave if there are no leftovers. I can also cook fried eggs with a sandwich press. Tinned fish can be a handy go-to if you need a quick meal – make sure it is in olive oil or brine and contains no seed oils. Again, make protein the hero of your meal – chicken, beef, pork, eggs, fish, or tofu if you are vegetarian.

Dinner is no different. When planning your meal, consider protein first. Most people are familiar with meat and three vegetables for dinner. Concentrate on above-ground vegetables if you want to reduce carb intake to lose weight or reverse some metabolic condition.

2. Add Healthy Fats

It's time to unlearn the outdated myth that eating fats makes you fat. In reality, our body needs fats, which consist of essential fatty acids, for bodily function. We need fat for hormone production. Fat is necessary for cell membranes. It is crucial for brain function. Our brain is primarily fat, around 60%. We can also burn fat for fuel.

This is particularly relevant when we reduce our carb intake, as we can switch our body's fuel system to burning fat. We can burn the fat we eat or the body fat we don't want. Wouldn't it be good to start burning that stubborn belly fat that won't go?!

Teaching your body to use fat as fuel is known as 'fat adaptation.' This helps stabilise energy, improve mood, sugar control, and aid long-term weight management and fat loss.

So, what does healthy fat look like? Think whole foods: avocado, olives, nuts, seeds, extra-virgin olive oil. Don't fear animal fats – the fat around the meat, chicken skin, pork crackling, duck skin or duck fat. Cooking with whole food fats, such as ghee, tallow, and butter, is all nutrient-dense and can be part of a nourishing diet.

As much as possible, you want to avoid the unhealthy, ultra-processed fats – in particular, the seed oils. These include vegetable oil, canola oil, sunflower oil, safflower oil, corn oil, cottonseed oil, rice bran oil, and margarine. These are extracted using chemical solvents, then refined, bleached, and deodorised at high temperatures.

The result is an inflammatory product high in Omega-6 and low in Omega-3. This disrupts the balance and contributes to oxidative stress, insulin resistance, inflammation, and chronic disease. There is emerging evidence linking high intake of these oils with heart disease, inflammation and even cancer.

Unfortunately, these oils are hidden everywhere in foods: in packaged snacks, biscuits, salad dressings, and mayonnaise. Restaurants like to cook and deep fry with these oils due to their low cost. Learning to read food labels is important – especially when recognising if these types of fats are hidden in processed foods.

3. Eat According to Your Carbohydrate Tolerance

How much carbs can you eat, or should you eat? You should eat according to your carbohydrate tolerance. This depends on many factors, such as activity level, insulin sensitivity, and metabolic health. If you are young, active, and don't have signs of insulin resistance, such as belly fat, skin tags, or raised blood insulin levels, you may be able to eat more carbs.

For example, my 16-year-old son plays sports daily and has a high activity level. He can tolerate more carbs without storing them all as fat. It's still best to choose whole, nutritious carbs such as fruit, root vegetables, and whole grains rather than refined carbs, processed foods, sugars, and snacks.

However, according to the *National Health and Nutritional Examination Survey* (NHANES) study in 2016, the estimate is that only 12% of the population in the USA meets the criteria for optimum metabolic health.[24] I believe Australia isn't far behind. Many individuals with a normal weight still do not meet the optimal criteria for metabolic health.

This highlights the importance of adopting a low-carb lifestyle, especially for those who are struggling with insulin resistance or want to lose weight. Even if you are metabolically healthy, reducing carbs can still be beneficial. Remember, carbs aren't essential for survival. We have around 100 years of experience in using ketogenic diets for people with epilepsy.[25] These people can control seizures by using the ketogenic diet.

To highlight our body functions without any problems, without carbs. We can use protein and fats for bodily functions and energy.

If you want to start cutting down on carbs, start by cutting down on simple carbs such as sugars, processed snacks, and sweets. If you can go the next step of cutting down bread, cereal, pasta, rice, and noodles, that would be even better. Reducing carbs can teach our body to shift from burning glucose to burning fat as fuel.

The principle of a ketogenic diet is drastically reducing carbs to less than 20 grams a day. This induces a metabolic state in which your body burns fat, producing ketones as an energy source.

For those who aren't ready for such drastic reduction, a low-carb diet, i.e., 50-100 grams of carbs, can still benefit your health and ease strain on your metabolism.

This means avoiding most breads, potatoes, snacks, sugar, biscuits, soft drinks, cakes, and rice. For fruit, I recommend not exceeding half a cup of fruit a day. Berries are lower-carb fruits and are typically the best choice.

If you like tracking, you can download apps such as *Carb Manager* or *Cronometer*. I don't suggest this to all of my patients as this complicates their lifestyle and makes it harder for them to adopt this diet. There are helpful food lists on websites. One of my favourite lists is Dr Peter Brukner's list from his book, *A Fat Lot of Good*.[26] Websites such as *Diet Doctor* and *Low Carb Down Under* also have abundant information.

You can download my free eBook from my website.

https://mlcclinic.com.au/free-resources/

I have also written a book called *Low Carb Made Easy*, which is a good companion to this book. It has lots of graphics, a food list, sample meal plans, and simple recipes for starting this lifestyle. You can purchase it from my website.

https://mlcclinic.com.au/online-course/

4. Add Salt and Flavours

When adopting a low-carb lifestyle, paying attention to your electrolytes, particularly sodium or salt, is essential. Especially in the first two weeks of transitioning to the low-carb diet, you shift from burning glucose to burning fat. Many people experience 'keto flu'. This can include symptoms such as headaches, fatigue, muscle aches, dizziness, and even cravings or withdrawal-like feelings.

One leading cause of these symptoms is loss of electrolytes, particularly sodium. When eating real food, there's not much salt. Another factor is that more salt is excreted in the urinary system when insulin is reduced.

During the initial period, you must get enough salt. Increasing salt intake can mitigate the keto flu symptoms. You can put more salt on food. You can drink electrolytes, ideally sugar-free. You can even put salt on your tongue, which sometimes helps some people reduce cravings. I would suggest aiming for 1-2 teaspoons of salt (5-10 grams) per day, but this may need to be adjusted based on individual needs and activity level.

In addition to salt, you can season your meals with flavours, herbs, and spices, such as rosemary, thyme, cumin, paprika, and turmeric. These not only enhance the taste of your food but also have anti-inflammatory effects that support your health. Adding healthy fats to your meals, such as olive oil, cheese, and avocado oil, can also help with satiety, increase nutrient density, and help you shift to fat-burning.

By ensuring you're consuming enough salt and flavouring, you'll help your body adjust more smoothly to the low-carb lifestyle and avoid many keto flu symptoms.

5. Eat Less Frequently

Your body triggers an insulin response to regulate blood levels every time you eat. Learning how to eat less frequently is another tool to improve insulin sensitivity and support fat burning. Because we often have abundant food and snacks, many people eat five or six times daily. We were also taught that snacking may increase metabolism.

Many also don't realise that drinks with calories, such as mid-morning milk coffee, will also trigger an insulin response and should be considered a snack.

You can start by practising time-restricted eating, which means eating three meals daily – breakfast, lunch, and dinner – without snacking in between. We should also remember to avoid drinks with calories between meals.

As your body adapts to burning fat for fuel instead of carbs, you may notice a decrease in hunger signals. At this point, when you are no longer hungry, you can delay your breakfast. Many can delay breakfast to 10am, 11am, or even noon, effectively transitioning to two meals daily.

This approach is called intermittent fasting. Some people extend their fasting window to 24 or 36 hours or even longer, offering additional benefits such as enhanced cell repair, autophagy (cleaning out damaged cells), reduced inflammation, improved insulin sensitivity and increased fat burning. Intermittent fasting has also been shown to reduce cancer risk and even help fight some cancers.

The Anti-Inflammatory Diet

This way of eating is actually anti-inflammatory, and that's a big deal, because chronic inflammation is at the root of many modern illnesses. Think of it like a slow-burning fire in the body that fuels disease.

Type 2 diabetes, for example, is linked to inflammation and insulin resistance.[27] High levels of insulin and glucose damage both large and small blood vessels, leading to complications like heart attacks, strokes, kidney disease, vision loss, and even limb amputations.

Heart disease is also driven by inflammation, primarily through atherosclerosis – the hardening and narrowing of arteries.[28,29]

Obesity isn't just about excess weight. Fat tissue acts like an endocrine organ, releasing inflammatory chemicals that raise the risk of diabetes, heart disease, and cancer.[30]

Alzheimer's disease is now being called 'type 3 diabetes' due to brain inflammation and insulin resistance, which prevent the brain from using glucose properly.[31]

Even **depression** and other mental health conditions are increasingly being linked to inflammation, poor brain energy, and mitochondrial dysfunction, not just genetics.[32]

Cancer, too, is being explored as a metabolic disease, with inflammation and mitochondrial damage playing a potential role in its development.[33]

And **non-alcoholic fatty liver disease** is now incredibly common, often driven by excess sugar, especially fructose, which over time can lead to liver scarring and cirrhosis.

This way of eating cuts out common triggers of inflammation, like sugar, seed oils, processed foods, and gluten. When combined with intermittent fasting, it can be a powerful tool for calming inflammation in the body. Many people start noticing improvements in symptoms like fatigue, bloating, aches, and pains even before they see any weight loss.

How to Personalise your Diet for Long-Term Success

Everyone is different. We come from different cultures, childhoods, and backgrounds. People have unique allergies, intolerances, tastes, family dynamics, work routines, activity levels, genetics, hormones, finances, medical conditions, medications, and personal values or beliefs.

That's why I don't believe in a one-size-fits-all approach like saying everyone must eat Keto or follow the same diet.

Personally, I'm Chinese and have cultural preferences in how I eat. I'm also quite active, doing strength training and running, and I have teenage boys who are constantly hungry, growing, and influenced by their peers. I also care for patients from many cultural backgrounds – some are vegetarian for religious reasons and have never eaten animal products.

I value these differences. My role is to help each person personalise their lifestyle so it works for them and sets them up for long-term success.

When a patient comes in, I take a thorough history of their diet and lifestyle. I ask how they normally eat and suggest small tweaks where needed. Some people need gradual changes, like adjusting one meal at a time. Others are ready to cut out bread, sugar, pasta, or snacks straight away.

Many need to boost their protein and healthy fats and realise that extra pasta or potatoes might slow down their progress. Some mums cook the same protein for the family, then swap the carbs – pasta for the kids, zucchini noodles for themselves. People who work outdoors may need to pack meals that suit their job, while others might grab takeaway or eat out. I help tailor strategies for any situation – whether it's prepping lunchboxes or choosing better options at a café, food court, or restaurant.

Your Prescription

o **Prioritise protein at every meal** – think eggs, meat, chicken, fish, tofu.

o **Add above-ground veggies** – leafy greens, broccoli, zucchini, etc.

o **Include healthy fats** – avocado, olive oil, butter, nuts, and oily fish.

o **Cut back on sugar and carbs** – bread, pasta, rice, cakes, and soft drinks.

o **Avoid seed oils and processed foods** – skip anything in a packet with a long list of ingredients.

o **Fasting is optional** – it can help some people, but it's not essential.

o **Customise to your life** – there's no one perfect diet. Fit it around your culture, family, work, and health needs.

Eat real food, nourish your body, and find what works for you.

Further Learning

Books

- *A Fat Lot of Good* by Dr Peter Brukner
- *A Big Fat Surprise* by Nina Teicholz
- *Why We Get Sick* by Dr Ben Bikman
- *The Obesity Code* and *The Diabetes Code* by Dr Jason Fung

People

- Gary and Belinda Fettke: check out Belinda's website and search interviewed done by both of them
- Dr Paul Mason: check out any interviews he has done
- Dr Lucy Burns and Dr Mary Barson: check out the *Real Health and Weight Loss Podcast* by *Real Life Medicine*

PART 2

The Movement Prescription

———————◆◇◆———————

CHAPTER 5

MOVEMENT: EXERCISE SMARTER, NOT HARDER

———————— ◆◇◆ ————————

"Happiness and fitness go hand in hand,
and exercise is one of the best ways to ensure both."
(George Washington)

Elizabeth's Story: Nordic Walking

Elizabeth just turned 70. She is keen to share her story with you. She has an incredible story of how staying active at the age of 70 can lead to a vibrant and fulfilling life.

She is a childcare worker, working two days a week. Outside of work, Elizabeth is committed to her health and movement. Not only does she follow a low-carb lifestyle, but she also prioritises movement. For the last four years, she's been working on staying active. She goes swimming four times a week – an activity she loves for its low-impact benefits. She maintains this lifestyle because she wants to avoid getting diabetes.

Three years ago, she discovered Nordic walking and immediately fell in love with it. Unlike regular walking, Nordic walking uses poles, which engage both the upper and lower body. This helps to build strength, stability, balance, and agility. She meets monthly with fellow walkers and eventually applied as a Nordic walker instructor to share the practice with others.

In addition to swimming and Nordic walking, Elizabeth also likes Pilates twice a week. Once a week, she meets with her 15-year-old grandson and enjoys walking and talking with him.

She recently shared how she challenged herself with a four-day hiking trip with her son and grandson at Wilsons Promontory. Her son was 43, and her grandson was 15. They trekked 19 kilometres through rugged terrain, carrying backpacks filled with tents, food, and gear. Elizabeth was proud to keep pace with the two younger men and wasn't left too far behind. She was proud of her strength, stamina, and adventurous spirit, showing that staying active into your seventies isn't just possible but empowering.

Anna's Story: Running at 59

Another fantastic story shared with me by a listener of my podcast is Anna, who is 59. She found a new lease of life and decided to take up running. She has a sedentary job, working in IT. Despite living on a farm with her husband, she sits in front of the computer most of the day. The only activities were walking up and down the hills of the farm. When she was younger, she enjoyed playing tennis, but exercise took a back seat until she began listening to the *Prescribing Lifestyle* podcast.

Inspired by my running adventures, Anna took up running – something she never thought she could do. Slowly, she built from 1 km to 2 km runs to confidently running 5km without stopping. Along the way, she remembered a book she had read earlier, *The Oxygen Advantage*.

In my podcast, I encourage my listeners to practice nose breathing instead of mouth breathing. Motivated by the podcast and the book she had read earlier; she began to build endurance running with her mouth closed. She even surprised herself by saying that she enjoys running.

Though weight loss wasn't her goal, Anna dropped 4kg, going from 70kg to 66kg. She proudly notes that she is the leaner sister compared to her identical twin.

With a renewed sense of strength and achievement, Anna is turning her focus to building muscle and plans to begin strength training next. Her journey is proof that it's never too late to start. Small, consistent changes can lead to remarkable transformation.

CHAPTER 6

THE EXERCISE MYTH: WHY YOU DON'T NEED TO 'BURN OFF' CALORIES

◆◇◆

As discussed in the previous chapter, our bodies are not bomb calorimeters. They aren't designed as simple mathematical equations of calories in versus calories out. The idea of eating less and moving more to lose weight is outdated. Our body is a complex system influenced by many factors, such as our age, activity level, gender, muscle mass, hormones, body composition, genetics, sleep, stress, and even Non-Exercise Activity Thermogenesis (NEAT).

The Myth of 'More is Better'

The common idea that 'the more you exercise, the more fat you burn' is misleading. I've had patients who diligently spent up to two hours a day doing repetitive exercises, hoping they could out-exercise their diet. The truth is, exercising more does not always equate to more fat loss. In fact, over-exercising can lead to increased hunger and increased inflammation. Your efforts could be counter-productive if you're not fuelling your body properly.

Additionally, excessive exercise can cause heightened stress, leading to elevated cortisol levels. This, in turn, can increase the risk of injury and chronic inflammation, making weight loss harder to achieve.

Your body responds to stress by holding onto fat as a survival mechanism, and chronic inflammation can impair metabolic function. It's crucial to remember that the **quality** of exercise is far more important than the quantity.

Finding Movement You Enjoy

It's essential to find the activity you genuinely enjoy, rather than focusing on burning calories you have eaten. I would encourage everyone to find a movement you like and look forward to, rather than treat it as a chore. This ensures long-term sustainability that you can keep going for many years into your age.

For example, if you thrive in a team environment, participating in team sports such as netball or football might be perfect for you. These activities not only encourage movement, but also connection and comradeship. Some people go to the gym to exercise and enjoy the social aspect and coffee connections after the gym class.

You can also have an accountability buddy who goes to the gym with you, making the experience more enjoyable and consistent.

For me, I started running to escape the constant demands of motherhood. I joined parkrun and even made some local friends with the same running interest – running allowed me to get out into nature. I also love seeing numbers. Seeing my 5km time reducing was another rewarding aspect.

Time-Efficient Workouts: HIIT

Many say they don't have time to exercise. They are busy going to work and looking after their children. Some exercises do not require a lot of time. Finding more efficient exercises may be beneficial for those who are time-poor.

High-intensity Interval Training (HIIT) offers a more time-efficient alternative to long, drawn-out endurance training. HIIT involves short bursts of intense exercise, followed by brief rest periods. For example, 30-second squats followed by 30 seconds of rest. Doing a few rounds of this can provide significant benefits compared to steady-state cardio in less time.

The advantages of HIIT are that it boosts cardiovascular health, improves strength, and increases fat burning – all in a shorter time. It's also easier to fit into busy lifestyles. [34,35]

When my kids were young, I used to wait for them to go to bed and do 10 minutes of body weight exercises in my lounge room. I would follow an app and do exercises including burpees, tuck jumps, and push-ups. After 10 minutes, it was enough.

This quick routine provided an energy boost, increased my metabolism, and improved my strength all within a short amount of time. It was also a great way to incorporate movement into my day with little need for space and equipment.

Strength Training: Building Muscle as We Age

Many women are unfamiliar with strength training. They are fearful of looking too muscular and bulky. Many do not understand the importance of building muscles as we age. Muscle and bone mass peak around the age of 30.

Quite often, after the age of mid-30s, our muscle and bone health declines. Without active training to build muscle and bones, we risk osteoporosis (loss of bone mass) and sarcopenia (loss of muscle mass).

Strength training helps reduce the risk of osteoporosis[36] and sarcopenia[37] and improves overall metabolic function, improving insulin sensitivity.

Strength training also reduces the risk of mental health disorders such as anxiety and depression[38] and improves brain health and cognitive function.

You can do strength training twice weekly for as little as 15 minutes.

Dr Ben Bocchicchio's *SMaRT Program*[39] is a great example of how efficient and time-effective strength training can be. *SMaRT* stands for Slow MAximum Response Training, which involves slow, controlled resistance exercises that maximise muscle engagement. Dr Bocchicchio claims that just 15 minutes, twice a week, of resistance training can lead to impressive results in fat loss and muscle gain.

The program is designed to be both efficient and effective, combining a controlled carbohydrate lifestyle to further optimise fat loss while building lean muscle mass. By focusing on slow, deliberate movements, *SMaRT* allows for maximum muscle recruitment without requiring hours of training.

Rest: Equally Important as Exercise for Building Muscle

It is equally important to rest as it is to exercise when it comes to building muscle. Muscle growth relies on adequate recovery after you've put your muscles through resistance training. When you exercise, you create small tears in your muscle fibres. These tears need time to repair and grow back stronger, which happens during your rest and recovery periods. Without sufficient rest, you risk overtraining, which can lead to muscle fatigue, injury, and even a decrease in performance.[40]

Ideally, with a strength-building program, strength training sessions should be spread out over the week, giving muscles the necessary recovery time. For example, you might do strength training on Monday and Thursday, allowing at least 48 hours of rest between sessions. On the other days, you can incorporate active recovery, such as yoga, stretching, walking, or swimming. These activities help keep your body moving without putting extra strain on your muscles, supporting both recovery and overall health.

Personally, I've found a routine that balances both strength training and cardio. I like to run three times a week and strength train twice a week, along with a weekly hike. I also ensure that I have at least one day of rest or lighter activity.

Monday and Wednesday are my strength training days, which give my muscles time to recover between sessions. Tuesday, Thursday, and Saturday are my running days, and on Sunday, I enjoy a hike to connect with nature and get some fresh air. On the days in between, I might go for a light walk or simply take it easy, depending on how my body feels.

This routine spreads out my exercises throughout the week, giving my muscles ample recovery time between strength training sessions while still maintaining a good level of activity. It allows me to stay consistent with my workouts without overtraining, helping me build muscle and improve my overall fitness.

Exercise for Long-Term Sustainability

Again, I realise everyone is different. We all vary in terms of age, activity levels, time constraints, family commitments, personal interests, and fitness goals. Some of us may have different medical conditions, physical abilities, or injuries, or may have had unique past experiences. My approach may not suit everyone, and that's okay.

What's important is finding something you enjoy, something that works for you, and fits into your lifestyle. Consistency is key. It's about integrating exercise into your life in a way that makes it sustainable, enjoyable, and prevents burnout.

When I started my exercise routine eight years ago, I joined the gym and took a close look at my schedule with my children's routines in mind. I realised I could commit to two gym sessions a week at 7pm and ask my husband to look after the kids for an hour. I scheduled those sessions into my diary as non-negotiable.

Over time, I added in some running – about 30 minutes while my kids napped in the afternoon. I gradually built up my exercise routine over a year or so, allowing my body to adjust and keeping my schedule flexible.

Finding the balance between exercise and other life demands took time, but by scheduling it into my routine and being consistent, I was able to make it part of my life.

CHAPTER 7

MOVING MORE, EXERCISING LESS

———————— ◆◇◆ ————————

Walking is one of the simplest and most underrated forms of movement. You don't need fancy equipment or a gym membership to start. It can be as easy as walking down your driveway to the mailbox or the end of your street. Maybe it's a 10-minute stroll around the block, or a 20-minute walk after dinner. Every step counts.

Even small changes – like parking a bit further from the shops or taking the stairs instead of the escalator – can make a difference over time. Maybe park your car 10 minutes away from work, so you end up with a 20-minute walk in a day.

Walking after meals can also be beneficial. Just a 10- to 15-minute walk after a meal can help with digestion, lower blood glucose, and increase insulin sensitivity.

Movement doesn't need to be structured or serious. **Dancing**, for example, is such a joyful way to move your body. Put on some music while you're cleaning, cooking, or hanging out with the kids or grandkids. Let go a little – have fun with it!

Stretching and **yoga** are also gentle yet powerful ways to move. It doesn't have to be a full hour-long session. Even a 10-minute flow in the morning or before bed can help improve circulation, increase flexibility, and relieve stress. You can search YouTube for free videos.

Gardening is another beautiful way to stay active. You're bending, lifting, reaching – and you're outdoors in the fresh air. You get a dose of sunlight (with sun protection, of course), and at the end of it, you have something to show for your efforts – flowers, herbs, or maybe even homegrown veggies.

Just **standing** more throughout the day can also support your health. You've probably heard the phrase, "Sitting is the new smoking." I bought a standing desk about a year ago, and it's been one of my best purchases. With just the push of a button, I can go from sitting to standing and keep my body from staying stagnant too long.

Movement can also be **social**. Go for a walk or hike with a friend, catch up on life while getting fresh air. It doesn't feel like a workout when you're chatting and laughing along the way.

One of my favourite weekend activities is parkrun. Originally started in the UK, it's now all around Australia. People gather every Saturday at 8am to complete a 5km course. Some run, others walk – it's totally up to you. I often walk it myself, and it takes me around 50 to 60 minutes. There are so many friendly faces, and you'll likely meet people who live nearby and become part of your community.

And finally, getting a **pet** can be an excellent motivation to move. Whether you're throwing a ball at the park or heading out for your daily walk, pets make movement more enjoyable – and their companionship is great for your mental health, too.

NEAT: The Unsung Hero of Metabolism

NEAT stands for Non-Exercise Activity Thermogenesis. It refers to the energy you burn through everyday activities that aren't structured exercise – things like walking, doing housework, playing with your kids, fidgeting, changing posture, standing, or pacing while on the phone.

You don't need to schedule a workout to benefit from movement. Simply weaving these activities into your daily routine can support better blood flow, help regulate blood glucose, and improve your overall health. Small changes, done consistently, can lead to big results.

The Ripple Effect: How Movement Fuels Your Whole Life

There's a growing body of evidence showing that physical activity can be just as effective as antidepressants in treating depression and anxiety, and without the side effects that often come with medication. Exercise helps to lower cortisol (the stress hormone) and boosts feel-good chemicals like endorphins, serotonin, and Brain-Derived Neurotrophic Factor (BDNF). In simple terms, movement helps create happy hormones.

Regular exercise also builds **resilience**. When you train your body to keep going even when it's tough, you're not just building physical strength – you're also strengthening your mental and emotional resilience.

It also supports better sleep. Movement during the day can help regulate your body clock, and if you're exercising outdoors, the exposure to natural sunlight boosts melatonin production, which aids restful sleep.

Exercising with others adds another layer of benefit. Group classes, walking groups, or community fitness events can foster social connection, improve self-esteem, and reduce feelings of isolation.

And let's not forget the metabolic perks – strength training in particular helps build muscle mass, which improves metabolism, supports mitochondrial health, and reduces insulin resistance.

Your Prescription

o **Find a movement you enjoy:** Walking, dancing, cycling, swimming, or Tai Chi
o **Schedule it:** Make it part of your routine and mark it in your diary
o **Exercise with others:** Partner up with a friend or family member for motivation
o **Start small:** Begin with just 10 minutes twice a week
o **Use resources:** Try apps, *YouTube* workouts, or online classes for guidance

Further Learning

Books

- *15 Minutes to Fitness DR Ben's SMaRT Plan for Diet and Total Health* by Dr Vincent 'Ben' Bocchicchio

People

- Dr Gabrielle Lyon, Functional Medicine Doctor and Founder of *Muscle-Centric Medicine*
- Dr Stacy Sims, Exercise Physiologist
- Dr Vonda Wright, Orthopaedic Surgeon, Author of *Fitness After 40, UNBREAKABLE* and *Younger in 8 Weeks*

PART 3

Sleep: The Ultimate Performance Enhancer

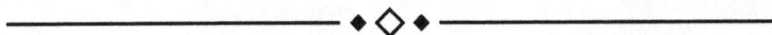

CHAPTER 8

SLEEP YOUR WAY TO A LEANER, HEALTHIER YOU: THE SECRET TO RESTORING AND REJUVENATING YOUR BODY

———————— ◆◇◆ ————————

"Sleep is the single most effective thing we can do to reset our brain and body health each day."
(Dr Matthew Walker)

Nola's Sleep Transformation

Nola is a 76-year-old woman who has been struggling with poor sleep for several years, especially after her husband was diagnosed with cancer. Around four or five years ago, she became a carer for her husband and often needs to stay up in the middle of the night caring for him.

With the added stress of managing cancer, she found her sleep to be broken. She would fall asleep at 10:30pm but wake up again after two to three hours, then lie awake for another two hours before eventually drifting off again.

Her sleep schedule became irregular. Some mornings, she would wake at 5:30am and other mornings, she would sleep until 8am or 9am to catch up. Despite her sleep challenges, Nola maintained a healthy, mostly low-carb diet in an attempt to stay healthy.

During our consultation, we focused on restoring her circadian rhythm. I explained the importance of consistent sleep and wake times. I encouraged her to get up at the same time, regardless of how good or bad her night's sleep was. I recommended getting outside for natural light to get her eyes exposed to sunshine.

Natural light exposure helps reset her internal clock. Midday sunlight exposure was already part of her routine as she enjoys gardening. I also encouraged an evening walk before sunset to further anchor her body's natural rhythm.

To help wind down, I suggested dimming artificial lights. She even bought blue-light-blocking glasses to wear while watching television. A two-to-five-minute breathing exercise at bedtime helped activate the parasympathetic nervous system and ease her into restful sleep.

A month later, Nola returned with a noticeable improvement in her sleep routine. Although she is still stressed about many aspects of her life, she feels she has the tools to manage her sleep far more effectively now.

Insomnia

When I was a teenager, staying up late was effortless. Like many other teenagers or young adults, I would go out to parties, stay up all night, sleep the next morning, and bounce back after a day or two. But that resilience doesn't last forever.

Everything changed when my son was born when I was in my 30s. My first son was a very unsettled baby for his first year of life. I experience tremendous sleep deprivation, reminding me of the importance of good sleep. My baby would wake every one to two hours, crying for either food or attention. I was suffering from sleep deprivation, living in a fog, exhausted, emotionally drained, and even feeling depressed.

I tried returning to work when he was six weeks old, aiming to work only half a day every fortnight. But even that became too much. Eventually, I had to take time off to recover as well as teach my newborn baby to sleep better.

As a GP, insomnia is one of the most common complaints I see. Many patients come in, hoping to be prescribed sleeping tablets as a quick fix. These patients may be going through a stressful period in their lives.

I also see many women in their perimenopause phase of life struggling with hot flushes and unable to sleep consistently.

Some women try everything to lose weight, reduce carbs, and exercise regularly. However, after further questioning, I found that they aren't prioritising their sleep. They may be staying up late, clinging to some quiet time after their children have gone to bed, or scrolling on their phones. Little do they know, not sleeping is a leading cause of failure to lose weight.

Sleeping tablets might offer temporary relief, but they have downsides. They don't provide natural, restorative sleep. They suppress deep and REM sleep stages essential for memory, repair, and emotional regulation. While they are helpful for short-term situations, long-term use can lead to dependence.

In this chapter, we'll explore why sleep is essential for energy and mood, metabolism, hormones, the immune system, and even weight loss. There's a lot more to unpack than just getting to bed on time.

Why Sleep Matters for Weight Loss

Lack of sleep doesn't just leave you tired and with brain fog; it can actually be a significant contributor to weight gain or make it hard to lose weight. There are a few mechanisms at play.

Sleep deprivation disrupts the intricate balance of your hunger and satiety hormones.

Ghrelin, the hormone that makes you hungry, increases appetite and rises when you don't sleep enough.

Leptin, the hormone that signals fullness, does not work correctly when you are sleep deprived.

This hormone imbalance often leads to cravings, particularly for high-sugar, high-fat comfort foods.

Lack of sleep also increases cortisol, the stress hormone, driving you to want more comfort food.

All these combined drive you to more emotional eating, reduced willpower and difficulty sticking to healthy habits.

This also creates a vicious cycle: Lack of sleep increases cravings and stress, which leads to poor food choices, weight gain, and further sleep disruption.

When you sleep, your body undergoes many functions, especially repair and restoration. During sleep, particularly deep non-REM sleep, your body repairs tissues, builds muscles, supports your immune system, and restores physical energy.

During REM sleep, your brain processes emotions, consolidates memories, and supports learning.

We need the right balance of different sleep stages.

At the cellular level, when you sleep, mitochondria, the powerhouses of your cells, undergo repair and recharge. They also do a 'clean-out' process, which helps your body use energy more efficiently and supports healthy metabolism. Sleep also stimulates growth hormone, which is important for muscle repair and fat burning.

Chronic sleep deprivation also increases inflammation, known to be a common contributor, if not the cause, of many chronic diseases, including heart disease, type 2 diabetes, Alzheimer's disease, mental health conditions, and certain cancers.

Finally, during sleep, your brain activates its clean-out system – the glymphatic system – which flushes out toxins and waste products that accumulate during the day. This process is crucial for brain health and cognitive function.

How Much Sleep Do We Really Need?

Sleep needs vary from person to person and across different age groups. If you wake up feeling refreshed and ready to start the day, you're likely getting enough sleep. However, if you wake feeling drowsy or find yourself yawning throughout the day, you may not be getting enough sleep, or the quality of your sleep may be suboptimal.

It's not just about the number of hours you sleep, but also about getting the right balance of sleep stages, including non-REM and REM sleep:

- Too little deep (non-REM) sleep can lead to fatigue and poor physical recovery.
- Too little REM sleep can impair memory, learning, and emotional regulation.

Sleep Needs by Age:
- Newborns, infants, and children require more sleep to support their rapid growth and development.
- Teenagers experience a natural shift in their circadian rhythm, often feeling sleepy later at night and needing to wake later in the morning. They still require eight to 10 hours of sleep to support brain development, physical growth, and emotional health.
- According to the *American Academy of Sleep Medicine,* adults generally need seven to nine hours of sleep per night.[41,42]

Sleep Statistics:
- Globally, one-third of adults sleep less than seven hours per night.
- In Australia, 40% of adults struggle to maintain a consistent seven to nine-hour sleep schedule.
- A global survey found that 62% of adults don't feel they get enough sleep, averaging 6.8 hours on weekdays and 7.8 hours on weekends.[43,44]

How to Get a Good Night's Sleep

Getting a restful night's sleep is one of the most potent and accessible forms of healing we have. Sleep is foundational for our immune system, mental health, metabolism, hormone balance, and emotional resilience. Yet, many people struggle to fall asleep, stay asleep, or feel refreshed in the morning.

The good news is that sleep is not just about luck – it's about creating the right conditions. Here's how you can take simple, practical steps throughout the day and night to promote deep, restorative sleep.

Set the Scene: Your Sleep Environment

Your bedroom should be a sanctuary dedicated to rest and recovery. Small changes can make a big difference:

- **Keep it dark, cool, and quiet** – Use blackout curtains, eye masks, and earplugs if needed.
- **Choose comfortable bedding** – A mattress that is too firm or too soft can disturb your sleep.
- **Cut off external light and noise** – Switch off unnecessary electronics and block outside disturbances.
- **Cooler is better** – A bedroom temperature between 16-20°C (60-68°F) is ideal for most people.
- **Declutter the space** – Hide clocks and screens. Avoid charging your phone near your bed. If possible, turn off Wi-Fi at night.

Throughout the Day: Lay the Foundation for Sleep

Your sleep quality at night is shaped by how you spend your day. Build healthy habits that signal to your body it's safe to rest:

- **Get moving** – Daily physical activity, like walking, yoga, or strength training, supports better sleep and mental health.
- **Seek natural light early** – Exposure to sunlight in the morning boosts melatonin production for the evening. Try sitting outside or going for a short walk.
- **Avoid stimulants** – Limit caffeine, nicotine, and alcohol, especially after lunchtime.
- **Watch your naps** – If you need to nap, keep it under 30 minutes and before 3pm.
- **Manage stress** – Practice deep breathing, mindfulness, or short meditations during the day.
- **Nourish your body** – Choose whole, unprocessed foods. Reducing sugar and refined carbs can support more stable sleep patterns.
- **Consider natural aids** – Supplements such as magnesium, zinc, melatonin, and calming herbs like chamomile, valerian, and lemon balm can help, though they're not for everyone.

Evening Wind-Down: Prepare for Rest
How you spend the evening sets the tone for the night:

- **Avoid vigorous exercise close to bedtime** – Finish workouts at least three hours before sleeping.
- **Eat early** – Avoid meals and large snacks within three hours of bedtime. Try time-restricted eating to help your digestive system rest, too.

- **Limit fluids** – Reduce fluid intake late in the evening to avoid waking up to go to the toilet.
- **Dim the lights** – Reduce artificial light exposure, especially blue light from screens. Try using blue light–blocking glasses or apps like *f.lux*.
- **Disconnect** – Avoid screens for at least one hour before bed.
- **Create a relaxing routine** – Whether it's brushing your teeth, meditating for two to five minutes, doing gentle yoga, or sipping a calming herbal tea, repetition trains your brain to wind down.
- **Avoid alcohol and smoking** – Both interfere with deep sleep.
- **Watch the sunset** – Nature's cue that it's time to rest.

While in Bed: Support Natural Sleep

Your bed should be reserved for two things: sleep and intimacy:

- **Avoid TV, scrolling, or reading in bed** – These can confuse your brain and delay sleep onset.
- **Don't clock-watch** – It increases anxiety and alertness.
- **Keep your phone out of reach** – Turn off notifications and avoid screens at night.
- **Can't sleep? Get up** – If you're tossing and turning, do something quiet and calming in another room until you feel sleepy again.

- **Optimal sleep window** – The best quality sleep typically happens between 10pm. and 2am. This is when your body clears sleep debt and starts deep repair.
- **Try breathwork** - Gentle breathing exercises such as slow nasal breathing or box breathing can calm your nervous system, reduce overthinking.

Morning Reset: Start the Day Right

Waking up well supports falling asleep again the next night:

- **Wake up at the same time daily, even on weekends** – Sleeping in disrupts your circadian rhythm.
- **Expose yourself to light** – Get outside or near a window within the first hour of waking. This helps reset your body clock and encourages healthy melatonin production for the night.
- **Create a positive start** – Practice gratitude, light stretching, or mindful breathing

Other Factors That May Affect Your Sleep

- **Diet** – Eating sugary or processed foods close to bedtime can cause blood sugar crashes and restlessness.
- **Light exposure** – Too little sunlight during the day or too much artificial light at night can throw off melatonin rhythms.

- **Preservatives and allergens** – Food additives or sensitivities can trigger inflammation or agitation, affecting sleep.
- **Nutrient deficiencies** – Low magnesium, vitamin D, or zinc may contribute to poor sleep.
- **Electromagnetic fields (EMFs)** – Turning off Wi-Fi or keeping devices out of the bedroom may reduce EMF exposure for sensitive individuals.
- **Health conditions** – Menopause, anxiety, depression, or chronic illness can disrupt sleep. These may need extra support and tailored strategies.

Sleep is not just rest – it's repair, growth, and protection. By building healthy daytime habits, creating a calming night-time ritual, and caring for your sleep environment, you can reclaim the quality sleep your body and mind truly need.

If you've tried the tips above and still struggle with sleep, learning about circadian health may be helpful. We'll explore this further in the next chapter.

CHAPTER 9

THE POWER OF YOUR INTERNAL CLOCK: HOW CIRCADIAN HEALTH TRANSFORMS YOUR SLEEP, MOOD AND METABOLISM

◆◇◆

It has been a fascinating journey learning about circadian rhythms. Initially, when I started studying lifestyle medicine, the focus was primarily on eating nutritious foods. However, as I delved deeper into the science of the circadian clock, I came to realise that it's not just about nutrition – it's also about energy. Our bodies not only get energy from food, but also from light. Every system in our body runs on internal clocks, and we are naturally programmed to function this way.

The body is controlled by a master clock, known as the Suprachiasmatic Nucleus (SCN), located in the hypothalamus of the brain. This clock regulates all body systems, including mitochondrial function, hormonal production, gut health, body temperature regulation, and thermoregulation.

When circadian health is disrupted – whether from jet lag, shift work, chronic sleep deprivation, or simply not getting enough sunlight – it weakens the SCN's ability to regulate sleep and metabolic processes. This dysregulation increases the risk of inflammation, mood disorders, weight gain, insulin resistance, Alzheimer's disease, and even cancer.

How to Improve Circadian Health

A regular sleep schedule is crucial. Waking up and going to bed at roughly the same time every day helps reinforce the body's natural rhythms.

Morning sunlight exposure plays a key role in resetting your circadian rhythm. Going outside first thing in the morning helps signal your body to produce melatonin at night, setting you up for restful sleep. A bonus is grounding – walking barefoot on the earth, which can help discharge excess electrical charge from the body. There's a lot more to discuss about grounding, but that's a topic for another day.

Taking short midday breaks outdoors – even just five to 10 minutes – can help regulate your circadian rhythm. Our ancestors spent much of their day outdoors, and sunlight exposure during the day aligns with our natural biological patterns. Evening walks, especially after dinner or near sunset, allow us to absorb gentle UV light, which further supports melatonin production and promotes better sleep.

In contrast, artificial lighting – often referred to as 'junk light' – lacks the full spectrum of natural sunlight and offers no health benefits. Exposure to artificial light at night (LAN) can disrupt the body's internal clock, reduce melatonin production[45], increase inflammation, and contribute to leptin and insulin resistance. Over time, this may raise the risk of chronic conditions such as weight gain, diabetes, and even cancer.[46,47,48]

To mitigate the effects of artificial lighting, dim the lights in the evening, especially in the few hours before bedtime. You can also wear blue light-blocker glasses to reduce the emission of blue light from screens. Alternatively, consider using bulbs that don't emit blue light in the evening.

Eating at consistent times helps regulate your circadian rhythm. People with circadian disruption may benefit from eating breakfast early in the day. Following an ancestral eating pattern – focusing on animal proteins, avoiding sugars, and processed foods – supports your body's natural rhythms. Also, try to avoid eating at least three hours before bedtime to allow your digestive system to rest in alignment with your circadian health.

There is a lot more to learn about circadian health. I encourage you to keep learning and explore what works for you.

Your Prescription

o **Set consistent sleep-wake times:** Stick to the same schedule daily, even on weekends.
o **Get morning sunlight:** Spend 10-15 minutes outside to reset your circadian rhythm, ideally as soon as you wake
o **Take midday breaks outside:** Expose yourself to sunlight during the day.
o **Walk after dinner or before sunset:** Boost melatonin production for better sleep.
o **Reduce artificial light:** Cut back on blue light exposure in the evening.
o **Practice grounding:** Walk barefoot on natural surfaces to connect with the earth.
o **Eat at regular times:** Avoid food three hours before bed.
o **Prioritise animal proteins:** Minimise sugar and processed foods for better sleep quality.

Further Learning

Books

- *Why We Sleep* by Matthew Walker

People

- Max Gulhane: his online courses and the *Regenerative Health* podcast

PART 4

Stress Management – Mastering the Mind-Body Connection

————————— ◆◇◆ —————————

CHAPTER 10

STRESS LESS, LIVE MORE: THE LIFESTYLE SHIFT FOR LONGEVITY

— ◆◇◆ —

Stress can come in many forms and from many different causes. In today's world, we live in a non-stop environment, constantly juggling demands. For instance, I have a busy household with two teenage boys who play sports – basketball and soccer. It can be stressful trying to find time to drive them to their games and practices.

On top of that, I work full-time and am focused on growing my low-carb clinic, while my husband runs a horticultural business and works six days a week to serve his customers. We both have elderly parents whom we care for. They are still in good health, but this can change in an instant.

Modern life often feels like a constant juggling act. We try to balance work, family, and personal time, but sometimes unexpected stressors arise. I remember when my father-in-law suddenly had a heart attack a couple of years ago on Easter Sunday. Fortunately, he survived but needed to undergo cardiac bypass surgery and later had a pacemaker inserted. It was a tough time for our family, but we got through it.

I have a patient around my age. She has three teenage boys who are very active in sports. She found herself overwhelmed, driving them to ten different sports activities in a week and feeling like she had no time for herself. She was constantly angry and grumpy, struggling to regulate her emotions. Her husband wanted to help but wasn't sure how.

To support her, I applied the skills I gained from Focused Psychological Strategies. Through a series of counselling sessions, we worked together to shift her mindset toward self-care. She began prioritising nutritious eating, incorporating protein into every meal, and started practising mindfulness more regularly. She also learned to delegate responsibilities to her husband and sought support from other mums to help with daily logistics.

Over time, she came to understand that she couldn't control everything and began placing her health, especially her lifestyle, at the forefront.

A couple of weeks later, she reported feeling more in control. The boys still needed to attend their sports, but she was able to manage her stress and adrenaline levels much more effectively. She found balance, and this helped her regain a sense of well-being amidst the chaos of her busy life.

I'm not a psychologist or a mindset coach, but I hope this chapter has helped you understand the science of stress and how deeply it affects your physical health. We're learning more every day about the powerful connection between the brain and the gut – mental stress can influence digestion, immunity, and overall well-being. I encourage you to explore different approaches to managing stress and discover what works best for you. Whether It's through mindset coaching, therapy, mindfulness, breathwork, meditation, or somatic practices, there are many tools available to support a more balanced nervous system.

How Stress Works: The Stress Response

Our bodies are equipped with systems designed to handle stress. When we encounter a threat or pressure, the hypothalamus in the brain communicates with the pituitary gland and adrenal glands.

In response, the adrenal glands release stress hormones like adrenaline and cortisol. These hormones trigger physical changes: our heart rate increases, breathing speeds up, and cortisol helps release glucose into the bloodstream for quick energy.

This acute stress response is helpful when it happens occasionally – it prepares us to respond quickly in challenging situations.

But in modern life, many people experience stress constantly, without a break. Many mums continually juggle work, looking after children, dropping off and picking up, after-school activities, financial stressors, looking after elderly parents, etc.

This ongoing, chronic stress can take a serious toll on the body. It can weaken the immune system, disrupt gut health, increase inflammation, and contribute to hormonal imbalances.[49,50]

Chronic stress has a profound impact on the brain. When cortisol levels remain elevated over time, it can interfere with memory, learning, and concentration. People may find themselves feeling forgetful, mentally foggy, or even experiencing symptoms of depression and anxiety.[51]

The amygdala – our brain's emotional control centre – also becomes overactive with chronic stress. This can heighten emotional responses, leading to increased irritability, anxiety, and sensitivity to future stressors.

Long-term stress also reduces neuroplasticity, the brain's ability to adapt and form new connections. This makes it harder to learn new skills, retain information, or adjust to change.[52]

Unfortunately, this often creates a vicious cycle. When we're stressed, we're more likely to neglect healthy habits – eating poorly, skipping exercise, and losing sleep, which only worsens our stress and its effects on the brain.

Sympathetic and Parasympathetic Nervous System

To truly understand how our nervous system works, we need to explore its two main branches: the sympathetic and parasympathetic nervous systems.

The sympathetic nervous system is responsible for our 'fight or flight' response. It is activated when we perceive stress or danger, prompting the release of hormones such as adrenaline and cortisol. These hormones mobilise glucose for energy, raise heart rate, and heighten alertness – vital for survival in our hunter-gatherer past, for example, when chasing prey. In modern times, this system is triggered by everyday stressors such as preparing for a job interview, giving a presentation, or having a difficult conversation.

While the sympathetic response is necessary in short bursts, chronic activation, which many people experience continuously, can have damaging effects on our health. Persistently high cortisol levels can impair memory and concentration, encourage fat storage around the abdomen, and elevate blood pressure and heart rate, increasing the risk of cardiovascular disease.

It suppresses the immune system, disrupts digestion by diverting blood away from the gut (leading to symptoms such as bloating, indigestion, or irritable bowel syndrome), and interferes with blood sugar control, raising the risk of insulin resistance and type 2 diabetes. It also impacts hormone balance, lowering libido, disrupting menstrual cycles, and reducing fertility, as the body deprioritises reproduction during perceived danger. Long-term stress is also linked to mood disorders such as anxiety and depression.

The parasympathetic nervous system, by contrast, helps restore balance. Often called the 'rest and digest' system, it supports essential functions like slowing the heart rate, lowering blood pressure, aiding digestion, and nutrient absorption, boosting immune function, and facilitating sleep, repair, and recovery.

You can activate your parasympathetic system through calming activities such as breathwork, meditation, gentle movement (like yoga or Tai Chi), spending time in nature, humming, gargling, or practising mindfulness.

In the next chapter, I'll explain how to use breathing techniques to engage your parasympathetic nervous system and help balance the stress response we face in daily life.

CHAPTER 11

FROM CHAOS TO CALM: STRESS-BUSTING SECRETS WITH BREATHWORK, MINDFULNESS, GRATITUDE AND JOURNALING

————————— ◆◇◆ —————————

"Your breath is medicine; free, instant and always available." (Unknown)

Susan, a 62-year-old woman, reached out to me after seeing my post about my offer on breathing retraining. She was going through a particularly stressful period in her life – having recently ended a relationship, acting as the primary carer for her elderly mother, and dealing with several physical injuries, including an injured elbow, an ankle injury, and knee pain.

When she sought help from her usual GP, she was offered antidepressants. To cope with her stress, she had also been relying on alcohol, consuming up to three bottles of scotch per week. During these times, she described feeling anxious, with erratic breathing and a racing heart.

Despite the challenges, Susan was already taking steps to support her health. She noticed drinking alcohol wasn't helpful, so she stopped just before coming to see me. She had also improved her diet by focusing on whole foods. She signed up to dance and went four times a week in an attempt to balance out her stress.

However, she knew her erratic breathing could be contributing to stress and anxiety and learning how to breathe better could be the key.

She came to see me for breathing retraining. I encouraged her to practise nose breathing at all times, including using a mouth tape during sleep. I also suggested she begin daily breathwork – ideally one to three sessions per day, lasting five to 10 minutes each. She joined several one-on-one guided breathwork sessions with me as well. She learnt to practice slowing down breathing, practising light breathing, and incorporating breathwork practices into her life.

After a month, Susan reported feeling significantly calmer. She was able to breathe through her nose consistently, both during the day and at night. Her breath-hold time, as measured by the Body Oxygen Level Test, had improved markedly. Most importantly, she felt empowered, equipped with a practical tool to regulate her nervous system during moments of stress and anxiety.

She described the experience as 'life changing.' Whenever something stressful occurs, she stops, slows her breathing, and reminds herself to 'Just breathe,' choosing to address the situation later. Through regular breathwork and mindful breathing, she learned to self-regulate.

Why I Swapped Prescribing Pills to Prescribing Breath: My Transformation into a Breathwork Facilitator

In 2023, I was invited by my friend Emma Martin, also known as *The Lazy Keto Mum*, to speak at a Keto retreat near the Gold Coast. It was an exciting opportunity to share my expertise on nutrition and metabolic health. The retreat combined a mini holiday with a speaking engagement and the chance to connect with like-minded individuals – a perfect getaway.

During this mini-holiday, I was doing what I love: running and listening to the *Huberman podcast*. On the same day, I stumbled across a new topic – the power of breath. As I listened to the other talks at the retreat, I attended one by Jarrod Stevenson on functional versus dysfunctional breathing. I had some basic knowledge from medical school on respiratory diseases, but this was something new. Jarrod recommended two books – *Oxygen Advantage* by Patrick McKeown[53] and *Breath* by James Nestor[54].

After the retreat, I took this as a sign to dive deeper into learning about breathing. I downloaded the audiobooks and was captivated. I wanted to understand more and began to explore how I could incorporate this into my practice. Eventually, I enrolled in the *Oxygen Advantage* facilitator course and, many months later, trained as a breathwork facilitator through *Breathless Academy* with Johannes Egberts.

The Birth of Breathe in Health

This journey has been transformative to my work as a GP. I began to notice that many patients weren't breathing properly. Children who breathe through their mouths instead of their noses are at higher risk of chronic cough, asthma, facial development issues, increased need for orthodontic treatment, and even anxiety. Simply switching from mouth breathing to nose breathing can significantly reduce snoring.[55,56] Learning to slow the breath can also help improve symptoms of depression, anxiety, ADHD symptoms, and even reduce the frequency of nightmares.[57,58]

Along the way, I launched my business, *Breathe in Health*. The name came from my 13-year-old son during a car ride when I shared my passion for helping patients improve their health through breathwork. I loved the name and immediately registered it as my new business.

I began working with patients one-on-one for breathing retraining and ran a four-week online course, teaching participants how to measure their breathing, practice simple breathing techniques, and regulate their nervous system. These tools can help them manage stress, improve sleep and ultimately, create healthier lifestyles.

Studies show that just a few weeks of practising slow, controlled breathing – typically around four to six breaths per minute – can lead to significant improvements in both physical and psychological well-being. Using slow breathing can activate the parasympathetic nervous system.[59]

This results in lower blood pressure, reduced resting heart rate, and decreased cortisol levels, the body's primary stress hormone. It also enhances heart rate variability (HRV), a key marker of nervous system balance and resilience. Often, these changes result in reduced anxiety, improved emotional regulation, and better sleep quality, making slow breathing a simple yet powerful tool for supporting overall health.[60,61]

Improving the way we breathe also influences many areas of health. Better breathing helps regulate cortisol and blood glucose[62], which in turn supports hormonal balance, appetite control, and weight management. It also enhances sleep, reduces cravings, and improves focus.

Because the body is interconnected, even small shifts in one area, like breathing, can create positive ripple effects across others. For instance, nasal breathing during physical activity increases aerobic efficiency and fat-burning potential, making exercise more effective and sustainable.

Today, I continue to work with patients one-on-one, helping them retrain their breathing. I host online courses and breathwork workshops, teaching participants to incorporate breathwork into their daily lives. I've created multiple guided breathwork recordings on *YouTube* and my podcast, and I've made some available on *Insight Timer*, a meditation and wellness app designed to support mental, emotional, and spiritual well-being. I've also been invited to lead breathwork sessions at various retreats.

Personally, I practise breathwork every morning without fail. Depending on how much time I have, I spend anywhere from 10-30 minutes using the *Insight Timer* app.

I also love participating in live breathwork sessions, which offer a different kind of energy and connection. They are like yoga classes, lasting around one hour, and practised lying down. Breathwork has profoundly impacted my own health, especially in helping me manage stress more effectively.

When I'm faced with something stressful, I consciously tune into my breath. One technique I often use is 'coherent breathing' – inhaling for a count of five and exhaling for a count of five. Simply shifting my focus from the stressful situation to the rhythm of my breath helps calm my mind and regulate my nervous system almost instantly. You can find a guided version of this breathwork in one of my episodes on the *Prescribing Lifestyle* podcast. (Episode 24)

Mindfulness and Meditation: The Art of Being Present

Mindfulness is the practice of being present and aware in the moment without judgment. It involves paying attention to sensations, thoughts, feelings, and surroundings. By focusing here and now, we let go of worries of the past and future. Mindfulness invites us to observe our bodily sensations and surroundings without labelling them good or bad.

Meditation is a practice that involves mindfulness or focused attention, often with a set time. It commonly focuses on the breath, bodily sensations, a body scan, or an affirmation to help centre the mind and promote relaxation.

Many people say they can't do meditation because they can't clear their minds. They believe they need a blank mind. This is actually not required. It's perfectly normal to have thoughts arise. The true practice lies in noticing those thoughts, acknowledging them gently, and letting them go. This is the practice of mindfulness. And the more you practice, the better it gets.

Mindfulness can also be brought to eating. We can remind ourselves to notice our bodily sensations if we are hungry or not. We can also practice looking at the food, seeing the shape, taste, and sensations when we eat. The more we practice, the more we learnt to tune into our hunger and fullness signals.

We learnt to eat when hungry, not out of boredom or comfort. We practice slowing down, chewing thoroughly, savouring flavours, and engaging all our senses. This awareness can help us make more intentional choices, enjoy our food more and reconnect with the act of nourishing our bodies.

Mindfulness can be integrated into everyday life, whether you are going for a walk in nature, noticing trees and birds, driving, seeing people walking on the streets, engaging in conversations at work or home, or playing with your children. Even online interaction can benefit from mindful awareness – pause before commenting.

Consider the acronym T̲H̲I̲N̲K̲:

- Is it T̲rue?
- Is it H̲elpful?
- Is it I̲nspiring?
- Is it N̲ecessary?
- Is it K̲ind?

Journaling: A Path to Self-Discovery

Journaling is a powerful tool for practising mindfulness and self-awareness. Writing regularly helps clarify your thoughts, untangle your mind, and process emotions. A journal is always there for you. There is no judgment. It is a safe space. It will listen and never talk back.

Journaling supports emotional regulation. Putting emotions into words helps you acknowledge and process them. There is no need to suppress. Naming and recognising the emotions can help you understand more about yourself and what is happening.

Journaling can also help with physical symptoms. You can document physical symptoms as you go along the weight loss journey, trying different foods. Keeping a food diary often raises awareness and identifies patterns of eating. Quite frequently, if you write down everything you eat, you will avoid grabbing the extra snack, as you don't want to be seen snacking mindlessly. This helps you keep accountable for yourself.

Keeping track of food and symptoms may help you identify symptoms, such as bloating, low energy, and poor sleep, that may be related to increased sugar intake. You can often reflect and remind yourself how good you felt when eating on track.

Regular journaling also strengthens cognitive function, supports clearer goal setting, and creates deeper connections with your values and vision.

Gratitude: A Daily Practice for a Fulfilling Life

Gratitude is a simple practice of thinking about what's good in your day, no matter how your day unfolds. There's always something to be grateful for, even on challenging days.

There are many ways to practice gratitude. Some people write in a journal. Some people start their day thinking about three things they are grateful for. My friend habitually asks her children to name one or two things they are thankful for at dinner time.

For me, I combine journaling with gratitude practice at bedtime. I keep a notebook by my bedside and write down at least three things I'm grateful for from the day, in point form. This takes only half a minute to write down before bedtime.

This practice was suggested to me by my health coach co-worker, Carla Veith-Carter. She recommends that at the end of each day, we actively reflect on the positive moments and highlight what went well.

Our minds tend to focus on the negative, and research shows that up to 80% of our thoughts can be negative. By consciously searching for the good, we can rewire our brains to focus on positivity instead of negativity.

Studies show that gratitude practice can significantly improve mental health, boost emotional resilience, enhance sleep quality, strengthen relationships, reduce stress, and lower cortisol and blood pressure. People who practice gratitude are also more likely to exercise, eat well, and attend medical check-ups.[63]

Your Prescription

○ **Breathe with purpose** – Spend five to 10 minutes daily practising coherent breathing (inhale for five, exhale for five) to regulate your nervous system and reduce stress. Do this once or twice, or up to three times a day.

○ **Prioritise true rest** – Make space for real downtime by pausing, doing nothing, and allowing your body and mind to recover.

○ **Move gently and often (preferably outdoors)** – Include daily movement like walking, stretching, yoga, or Tai Chi to support physical and emotional balance.

○ **Create healthy boundaries** – Limit multitasking, take breaks from screens, and confidently say no when needed to protect your energy.

○ **Stay connected** – Reach out to friends, enjoy shared meals, or engage with a supportive community to strengthen emotional well-being.

○ **Use calming tools that resonate with you** – Choose practices like meditation, journaling, somatic work, or breathwork techniques that help soothe your system.

○ **Reflect and reframe your day** – End your day by practising gratitude or noting three positive moments to promote a more balanced perspective.

Further Learning

Books

- *Oxygen Advantage* by Patrick McKeown
- *Breath* by James Nestor

PART 5

Community and Mindset – the Missing Ingredients for Lasting Success

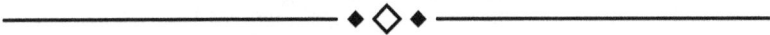

————— ◆◇◆ —————

CHAPTER 12

MIND OVER METABOLISM: REWIRING YOUR BRAIN FOR SUCCESS

————————— ◆◇◆ —————————

"Old habits are hard to break because the subconscious mind resists change, even when it's for the better." (Anonymous)

I'm going to share my own experience of a bad habit. I don't like admitting it, but I have a bad nut-eating habit. This might sound familiar to those of you who want to have a drink of alcohol before dinner.

At 5pm, after a busy day at work, I come home, and whilst cooking dinner, I like to have a snack of nuts. It could be macadamia nuts or cashews. It was my way of unwinding after a busy day at general practice. I thought I'd reward myself. But as soon as I have a handful, I cannot stop. Before I knew it, I might have had half a bag of them. Sometimes I eat so much that I don't even feel like having dinner. I thought about the nuts before I got home, even while in the car on the way home.

This behaviour became a habit, and often, when I reached for the nuts, I wasn't even thinking about it. I'd finish a small bowl, then pour a few more, and then a few more again.

Learnt Behaviour and Habit Formation

For us to understand habits, we need to know how our mind works – many of the behaviours we do as adults are ingrained when we were children. Before the age of eight to ten, we absorb experiences, often unconsciously. These experiences are stored away in our brain, like a filing cabinet. We usually operate mindlessly, pulling out each file from the filing cabinet without thinking. We repeatedly do the same thing because our unconscious mind operates without thinking.

For example, if we were taught as children that when we are feeling down or hurt, Mum would cheer us up with food, maybe something sweet like ice-cream. Over time, we may understand to self-soothe, eat something sweet, or it's a treat for us, especially when feeling low.

This is not an effective coping mechanism because we haven't dealt with emotions but pushed them down with something comforting. As we age, we unconsciously reach for comfort food to deal with emotions. This learnt response is automatic, and we may not even realise until we stop and pay attention.

The Psychology of Habit Change

First, it's important to understand that much of our behaviour is guided by the unconscious mind. We are often driven by subconscious beliefs and emotional triggers that stem from early life experiences. As a result, our minds tend to operate on autopilot. Over time, many of us learn to self-soothe by avoiding discomfort, developing habitual behaviours that serve as coping mechanisms.

Recognising that we've entered a habit loop – a cycle of trigger, routine, and behaviour – is the first step toward change. Awareness allows us to identify these patterns and begin the process of transformation.

Building this awareness is crucial.

Cultivating a positive self-image, practising self-care, and embracing self-compassion can reinforce our ability to break free from old habits.

Consider habit formation akin to walking on a trail. Established paths are easier to navigate, but forging a new route requires effort and repetition. Clear the undergrowth, then tread the path consistently, and then this becomes a known pathway and easier to navigate.

To disrupt our ingrained habits, we need to understand their origins, often embedded in our subconscious mind from childhood. First, we are aware of what's happening in our mind, i.e. mindful awareness. Next, a conscious decision to avoid the old habit, combined with practising new behaviours, helps to form new neuropathways.

This process is challenging. Seeking support from professionals, such as psychologists, psychotherapists, or health coaches, helps change habits. Additionally, having an accountability buddy or partner can provide lots of encouragement and motivation.

Breaking the Nut-Snacking Habit: A Personal Journey

I've realised that my evening nut-eating habit evolved through habitual behaviour. This is no longer serving my well-being. At the end of a demanding day, I often find myself seeking comfort, reaching for the nuts was an automatic, unconscious behaviour.

To address this, I've made a conscious decision to stop stocking nuts in my pantry, removing the trigger for this unconscious behaviour. In place of this habit, I am cultivating new routines that provide relaxation without relying on food.

Around 5pm, instead of heading to the pantry, I decided I could sit outside and pat my dog. I might take a few slow, mindful breaths before commencing dinner preparations. Alternatively, I might play a calming YouTube video or listen to a podcast while cooking. These intentional practices help me remain present and grounded and reduce the likelihood of mindless snacking. By understanding my triggers and implementing mindful strategies, I work towards healthier habits that align with my overall well-being.

It's essential to practice self-compassion. If you slip back to old habits, remember you were ingrained in this for a long time. Our minds have been conditioned over the decades. Changes take time. Don't beat yourself up if you slip into these old ways. Try to practice being more conscious in the future to avoid slipping up again.

In the following chapter, we'll explore how the power of community and support can help us sustain our journey towards lifestyle change.

Your Prescription

o **Recognise:** Take a moment to notice which habits are helping you and which ones are holding you back.

o **Decide:** Consciously choose the habits you want to build. Focus on small, meaningful changes that support your well-being.

o **Get support:** Change is easier with help. Reach out to a friend, coach, or professional if you need guidance or accountability.

o **Break through:** When old patterns surface, pause and ask: What's the most caring thing I can do for myself right now? Choose the action that aligns with your best self.

Further Learning

Books
- *Atomic Habits* by James Clear

CHAPTER 13

THE POWER OF CONNECTION: WHY COMMUNITY IS MEDICINE

— ◆ ◇ ◆ —

"Alone, we can do so little; together, we can do so much." (Helen Keller)

The Silver Linings of COVID-19: Rediscovering the Power of Community

In the years 2020 and 2021, Melbourne became the world's most locked-down city. My friends, family and I experienced firsthand the profound effects of COVID-19 and the global pandemic. The pandemic isolated us in a way we never experienced or anticipated. Socialising became difficult. We were restricted in whom we could visit. We couldn't go to school or work, and there was no social life. Many were forced to work from home.

As a GP, I noticed a rapid rise in mental health consultations, especially among certain vulnerable groups. These include with teenagers, the elderly, those living alone with chronic illnesses or those with existing mental health conditions.

While we adapted through virtual communication, it couldn't fully replace the value of face-to-face connections. The pandemic made us understand how essential community and social support are for our mental health and our sense of belonging.

The Power of Support

I have witnessed that those in the low-carb community especially need more community and social support to sustain this lifestyle. Practising low carb is different to the usual population. Most friends and families may not understand the rationale for not eating everyday foods. It's different from the conventional dietary advice most people follow.

Some of us are doing this alone within our families. Many women may not be supported by their husbands or children. I, myself, am the only person in my household following a low-carb lifestyle. It can feel isolating when those closest to us don't share the same values or health goals. Dining out with friends can also be challenging. It's difficult for outsiders to understand our food choices. It's in these moments that a supportive community becomes especially important.

Setting up Online Low-Carb Communities

Early in my journey with the *Melbourne Low Carb Clinic*, I recognised the importance of community support. A few years ago, health coach Tracey McBeath invited me to help set up the *Low Carb Melbourne Facebook* group. Alongside others, including Gillian Harvey, Helena Kastanis, and Darren Graham, we continue to manage the group to support individuals exploring and living a low-carb lifestyle.

Gillian Harvey has done lots of work organising monthly lunch gatherings at a local cafe that offers a low-carb-friendly menu. This provided the community a space to gather, connect, catch up and encourage each other.

To extend this support, I founded the *Melbourne Low Carb Clinic Free community*. I share recipes and meal ideas and encourage members to share their highs and lows. I also share many resources and insights to help members with their lifestyle changes.

Many similar supportive social media groups and communities share the goal of helping people succeed with lifestyle changes.

I also run a paid membership program called *Low Carb Pro*, which provides fortnightly *Zoom* gatherings and accountability support. I give a talk each session on a specific topic, often suggested by members. It's been incredibly rewarding to witness the strength of women supporting each other in a safe, understanding space.

Being surrounded by others who understand and empathise with your journey reduces feelings of isolation, anxiety, and stress. It reminds us that we are not alone. Community helps us stay accountable. We celebrate each other's wins and support each other on lows. We also grow by learning from each other through new perspectives, ideas, and strategies.

Ultimately, humans are wired for connections. Being part of a supportive community strengthens the sense of belonging, helping us feel seen, heard, and valued. In addition to online groups and gatherings, I have organised and attended various low-carb dinners, conferences, and supportive events that further strengthen the sense of community among like-minded individuals.

The Power of a Health Coach

Many studies show that individuals working with a health coach as part of a weight loss program experienced more significant weight loss compared to those who didn't have a coach. Health coaching helps individuals stay accountable, establish healthier habits, and overcome barriers to long-term success.[64]

Other studies have also shown that having a health coach can help patients effectively manage chronic diseases like diabetes, hypertension, and heart disease. Health coaches can also enhance physical activity and psychological and emotional well-being.[65,66,67]

At the time of writing, I collaborated with health coach and nutritionist Carla Veith-Carter from *Keto By Design*. We started working together at the beginning of 2025 and designed a program called *The Metabolic Makeover Program*.

It is a packaged program including two consultations with me, the GP, and four consultations with Carla, for coaching and accountability. We also provide *the Complete Guide to Low Carb Online Course* and the *Low Carb Pro* membership program. We are hoping participants will have ongoing support over many months, establishing and consolidating positive lifestyle changes.

Your Prescription

o **Surround:** Surround yourself with like-minded individuals who share your values and goals.
o **Connect:** Seek out or create safe, supportive spaces where you can connect, share, and grow.
o **Seek support and accountability**: Let others walk beside you – support and accountability make change more sustainable.
o **You are not alone:** Remember: healing, growth, and transformation are easier when we're not alone.

PART 6

Understanding Addiction – the Brain, the Behaviour, the Struggle

————————— ◆◇◆ —————————

CHAPTER 14

MANAGING ADDICTION: BREAKING FREE FROM WHAT HOLDS YOU BACK

——————◆◇◆——————

"Addiction isn't about a lack of willpower.
It's about your brain being hijacked by substances
that manipulate your neurochemistry."
(Dr Anna Lembke)

John's Story: From Alcohol Addiction to Recovery

John is a 60-year-old organisational psychologist, a high-functioning professional working for corporate companies. He has generously agreed to share his story of alcohol addiction – a struggle that almost cost him his life. Despite his professional success and discipline, John found himself helpless in the face of alcohol misuse. He has now been sober for the past 14 months.

John was referred to me by a health coach who advocates for a low-carb lifestyle after he was newly diagnosed with type 2 diabetes. He embraced the lifestyle, reduced his carbohydrate intake, lost weight, and improved his blood sugar control. As a result, he was able to reduce some of his medications – a fantastic achievement.

However, alcohol remained an area he couldn't control.

Looking back on his life, John recalls a family history of alcohol addiction – his father and grandfather were both alcoholics. He began drinking at age 14 and has always drunk to excess. Yet for decades, he maintained the discipline to limit his drinking when needed. During periods of intense work or study, he was able to stop. He built a successful career in the corporate world and maintained his physical health through regular exercise, trying to offset the effects of alcohol.

However, the COVID-19 pandemic marked a turning point.

Working from home and experiencing boredom and isolation, John's drinking escalated. He identified two key triggers for his drinking: times of celebration and times when things went wrong. Eventually, his drinking became nightly, up to a bottle of vodka each evening. He felt utterly out of control.

Alongside his addiction, John struggled with anxiety, depression, and possibly undiagnosed ADHD. He would sometimes binge over a three-day period in an attempt to obliterate his emotional pain.

A little over a year ago, alcohol nearly took his life.

Feeling helpless and broken, unable to control himself, John made a suicide attempt. He took all the sleeping and anxiety medications he had at home – some prescribed to him, and some stolen from his wife. Miraculously, his wife came home two hours earlier than expected, found him unconscious, and called an ambulance. Emergency services were able to revive him, and he was transferred to the hospital, then to alcohol rehabilitation.

That event changed his life.

Since that near-death experience, John has committed to sobriety. He acknowledges it hasn't been easy. He continues to experience cravings and must actively work to stay on track. He now attends *Alcoholics Anonymous* meetings two to three times a week, has a sponsor who has been sober for 23 years, and regularly works with a psychotherapist on mindset and emotional health. He also sees me for ongoing GP support.

John says that one of the most powerful tools in his recovery has been reconnecting with his sense of spirituality – not in a religious sense, but through what he calls 'humanistic values': honesty, respect, kindness, love, and tolerance.

What is Addiction?

Addiction is a chronic, relapsing brain condition. It involves compulsive use of a substance or engagement in a behaviour, where the brain continues to seek reward despite harmful consequences.

In the modern world, addiction often involves substances such as nicotine, drugs, and alcohol. It can also include behaviours like screen use and gambling. These substances and activities increase dopamine levels in the brain, triggering the brain's reward system. In recent years, sugar and food addiction have increasingly been recognised as legitimate conditions.

As use continues, the brain develops tolerance, meaning more of the substance is needed to achieve the same effect. This often leads to dependence, where the person needs the substance just to function normally. People with addiction commonly experience a loss of control, intense cravings, continued use despite knowing the harm, and withdrawal symptoms when they try to stop.

Your brain is essentially hijacked by the substance or behaviour. You're hooked by the surge of dopamine it releases, reinforcing the cycle of addiction.

Peter's Story: Sugar Addiction

Peter is a 52-year-old construction worker who does shift work, often during the night. He is happy for me to share his journey of overcoming sugar addiction, which he managed to control through adopting a carnivore lifestyle.

Peter has two sons – one aged 25 from a previous marriage, and another who is five years old – as well as a two-year-old grandson. He is now working hard to teach his young children and grandson about the dangers of sugar addiction, hoping they won't follow in his footsteps.

From a young age, Peter was constantly exposed to sugar. His grandmother owned a cake shop, and his mother ran a cake decorating business. He grew up surrounded by sweet foods and regularly helped his mother decorate cakes, piping icing onto them.

He remembers waking up at 4am to do paper rounds from the age of 11 and eating enormous breakfasts – 15-20 *Weetbix* topped with milk, cream, and sugar. His home was always filled with biscuits, cakes, and snacks.

He would often eat six to ten times a day or even more, including croissants, sugar buns, apple scrolls, cheesy pasta, and other refined carbs.

His father prepared balanced dinners of meat and three vegetables, usually followed by a sugary dessert. However, Peter had an enormous appetite, and by his early teens, he had already learned to cook. He would make himself extra meals with bread or pasta to fuel his growing body and athletic training.

Peter trained intensively in professional tennis and other sports, which he believed justified his large energy intake. His physical demands, growing body, and shift work lifestyle contributed to constant sugar cravings and disrupted circadian rhythms. He still maintains an athletic lifestyle, including mountain biking and rock climbing.

At the height of his sugar addiction, Peter described operating on 'autopilot'. He recalls once driving to the country to visit his now-second wife and not remembering parts of the journey – completely disconnected and distracted.

A few years ago, his wife began exploring the Keto lifestyle to improve fertility. Peter joined her and eventually transitioned fully to a carnivore diet. The results were dramatic. His mental clarity significantly improved. He remembers driving back from a three-day training in

Sydney to Melbourne and still feeling sharp and alert – a stark contrast to how he used to function on a sugar-heavy diet.

Peter says the carnivore lifestyle has changed his life. He is determined never to return to his old eating habits and is now highly conscious of his children's and grandson's health, focusing their diets primarily on protein.

On an unrelated note, Peter also suffered from chronic asthma and severe snoring. When I offered functional breathing training, he volunteered. After three days of practising nose breathing and following my advice, his snoring dramatically reduced. He joked that I 'saved his marriage' as his wife could finally sleep comfortably beside him again.

The Addicted Brain: Hijacked, Hooked and Held Hostage

Addiction is a complex condition with many contributing factors. As shown in the above two stories, there may be a genetic predisposition or childhood experiences that can significantly increase the risk of developing addiction later in life.

Some individuals have a history of childhood trauma; Adverse Childhood Experiences (ACEs) are common.

In studies that look at ACEs, we understand that they can have profound, long-lasting effects on physical and mental health across a person's life. It can stem from abuse, physical, emotional, or sexual. It can be from neglect, physical or emotional. It can also be from household dysfunction, such as parental substance abuse, domestic violence, parental separation, or divorce.[68,69]

Many individuals who suffer from addiction describe a profound loss of control and willpower. They feel their brain is hijacked, hooked, and held hostage. They are unable to control their brain. Telling someone who suffers from addiction to 'just stop' is not only unhelpful but can be deeply invalidating. Addiction is not a choice; it's a brain condition that makes stopping impossible.

Certain triggers, for example, emotional distress, fatigue, stress, sleep deprivation, and even joyful celebrations, can trigger addiction. People feel depressed, hopeless and resort to self-medicating with the very substance or behaviour they are trying to avoid. This perpetuates into a cycle of addiction, shame, guilt, and relapse.

Recognising Addiction: Screening Tools

Recognition is the first step to change. Screening tools can help individuals and clinicians identify patterns of addiction.

CAGE Questionnaire (for alcohol use):[70]

- **C** – Have you ever felt you should **Cut down** on your drinking?
- **A** – Have people **Annoyed** you by criticising your drinking?
- **G** – Have you ever felt **Guilty** about your drinking?
- **E** – Have you ever had a drink first thing in the morning to steady your nerves or get rid of a hangover (**Eye-opener**)?

Two or more 'Yes' answers suggest clinically significant alcohol use and may indicate dependence or misuse.

UNCOPE Questionnaire (adapted for food addiction):[71]

- **U** – **Unplanned use**: Have you spent more time than intended obtaining or eating certain foods?
- **N** – **Neglected**: Have you ever neglected your responsibilities because of food?
- **C** – **Cut down**: Have you ever wanted to cut down or stop eating certain foods, but found you couldn't?
- **O** – **Objected**: Has anyone ever objected to your eating habits or expressed concern?
- **P** – **Preoccupied**: Have you used food to escape from emotions, stress, or problems?
- **E** – Have you ever had a drink first thing in the morning to steady your nerves or get rid of a hangover (**Eye-opener**)?

Two or more 'Yes' answers may indicate problematic food-related behaviours or food addiction. While this tool is not diagnostic, it helps flag loss of control, cravings, and the impact on daily function.

Unhooked: Rewiring the Brain from Drug and Alcohol Dependence

There is extensive research and well-established treatment pathways for drug and alcohol addiction. As a GP, I'm often the first point of contact for someone seeking help. My role typically involves initiating the process and referring patients to appropriate drug and alcohol treatment services in the community.

Treatment options vary depending on individual needs and can include both public and private programs. Some patients may benefit from inpatient or outpatient detox services, while others are better suited to community-based support. Many community health centres also offer specialised drug and alcohol counselling.

Detoxification and withdrawal management may be necessary, either as an inpatient or at home with appropriate supervision. Medications are sometimes prescribed to ease withdrawal symptoms and support recovery during this phase.

Psychological support is a key part of recovery. Therapies such as Cognitive Behavioural Therapy (CBT) and Motivational Interviewing (MI) are commonly used and can be highly effective. For those struggling with food addiction or disordered eating, working with a psychologist who specialises in eating disorders can be particularly helpful.

Peer support is another essential component. Groups like *Alcoholics Anonymous* (AA) or other community-based recovery programs provide connection, accountability, and shared wisdom. Support from family and friends is also vital – it often makes the difference between success and relapse.

Finally, I always encourage patients to make foundational lifestyle changes that support long-term recovery. This includes:

- Prioritising **whole-food nutrition** (low sugar, low processed foods)
- Engaging in regular **exercise**
- Establishing a consistent **sleep routine**
- Practising **stress management** through techniques like mindfulness, breathwork, or journaling

Healing from addiction requires more than willpower – it's a multi-layered process that supports the mind, body, and spirit. With the right team and tools, it's entirely possible to get unhooked and reclaim a healthier, freer life.

A Compassionate Approach to Food Addiction

Sugar and food addiction are not as widely recognised as substance addictions, and there are far fewer support programs available. But in my view, sugar and food addiction should be taken just as seriously. When patients come to see me, I treat it as I would any other illness, without judgment or stigma.

Addiction is not a failure of willpower. Many patients struggling with sugar or food addiction say it feels even harder to overcome than drugs or alcohol, because we need food to survive. The goal isn't abstinence from all food but learning to break free from the cycle of craving, loss of control, and emotional eating.

Step 1: Awareness and Naming the Problem

The first step in healing is awareness. Naming it 'addiction' helps people recognise that their experience is valid and that help is available. It also opens the door to recovery by reducing shame and allowing them to approach it as a health condition, not a personal flaw.

Step 2: Environment Preparation

Preparation is key. This involves clearing the home of trigger foods, such as sugar, biscuits, chips, or ultra-processed foods. At the same time, stocking up on nourishing foods – nutrient-dense meals rich in protein and healthy fats – is essential. These help keep blood sugar stable and reduce the likelihood of cravings.

Many individuals with sugar or food addiction are paradoxically overfed yet undernourished, consuming large quantities of low-nutrient foods while lacking essential vitamins and minerals.

Step 3: Support and Accountability

Support and connection are crucial for those with food addictions. Just like with alcohol or drug addiction, the community is vital. Whether it's family, friends, a health coach, or an online support group, having someone to talk to when cravings hit can make all the difference.

Daily accountability, like text messages from a coach or regular check-ins, can be incredibly helpful in moments of vulnerability.

Step 4: Strategies to Manage Cravings

Education about craving management is essential. Patients need to feel empowered with practical tools. One such tool I often recommend is the *DDD Method* created by clinical psychologist, Victoria Webster:

- **Delay**: Pause for 25 minutes. Cravings tend to pass, especially when the brain is redirected.
- **Distract**: Engage in an activity – go for a walk, call a friend, or get busy with something else.
- **Decide**: After delaying and distracting, decide whether to eat the food. Ask yourself:
  - Will this nourish or punish me?
  - How will I feel tonight or tomorrow?
  - Is this in line with my health goals?

Step 5: Practising Self-Compassion

Relapse can be part of the process. What matters is how we respond. Self-compassion is critical – beating yourself up only fuels the cycle. Instead, support yourself like you would a loved one. Get back on track, reflect on what triggered the slip, and keep moving forward.

Lifestyle Foundations for Recovery

Beyond food, other lifestyle pillars can support addiction recovery:

- **Low-Carb/Ketogenic Diets**: These can reduce hunger and cravings by increasing satiety through ketones.
- **Meal Timing**: Start with structured eating (e.g., three meals daily), then reduce to two or one meal per day as hunger stabilises.
- **Movement**: Begin with 20-30 minutes of daily walking, and progress to light cardio or

strength training for mental well-being and time structure.

- **Stress Management**: Mindfulness, breathwork, and meditation help calm the mind and reduce overwhelm.
- **Prioritise Sleep**: Good sleep regulates hormones, improving mood and hunger control.

Food addiction recovery is possible – but it takes more than willpower. It requires understanding, preparation, support, and compassion. As clinicians, friends, or loved ones, we can offer a safe space for healing and the tools to truly set people free.

Across the globe, several specialists are working toward gaining recognition for food addiction as a legitimate condition. Several studies have explored the use of low-carbohydrate or ketogenic diets as a therapeutic approach, and early results show promising positive effects in reducing addictive eating behaviours.[72,73]

Your Prescription

o **Awareness**: Recognise the signs of addiction and be honest with yourself.
o **Education**: Learn how addiction affects your brain and behaviour.
o **Support**: Reach out for help; recovery is stronger with connection.
o **Environment**: Remove triggers and set up your space for success.
o **Action**: Take small daily steps toward your goals – you're in control.
o **Self-Compassion**: Be kind to yourself; setbacks are part of the journey.

Further Learning

People:
- Dr Joan Ifland, a world-leading expert in processed food addiction
- Bitten Jonsson, a nurse with over 40 years of specialisation in the treatment of sugar and carbs addiction

PART 7

Going Forward

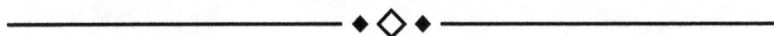

———————— ◆◇◆ ————————

THE LIFESTYLE PRESCRIPTION

YOUR PLAN FOR LASTING WEIGHT LOSS AND VIBRANT HEALTH

———————◆◇◆———————

"The lifestyle prescription is the most powerful tool we have for prevention and healing — by changing our habits, we can transform our health, reclaim our vitality, and unlock the potential for a longer, more fulfilled life." (Unknown)

Tracking What Matters: Using Biomarkers to Support Metabolic Health

One of the most valuable tools I use in assessing metabolic health is blood testing. These tests help tell the story of how your body is functioning, right down to the mitochondria, the tiny powerhouses in your cells. Together, these biomarkers provide a clear picture of your metabolic health and guide our treatment decisions.

Here are some of the tests I commonly request:

- **Full Blood Examination (FBE)**
  is a test that checks haemoglobin, white cell count, and platelets to assess for anaemia, infection, or other blood disorders.
- **Urea, Electrolytes, and Creatinine (UEC)**
  assesses kidney function and electrolyte balance, including sodium, potassium, and chloride.
- **Liver Function Tests (LFTs)**
  measure liver enzymes such as ALT, GGT, ALP, and AST. Elevated levels can indicate liver inflammation or fatty liver, which is often caused by excess sugar or fructose intake.
- **Inflammatory Markers: CRP and ESR**
  C-Reactive Protein (CRP) and Erythrocyte Sedimentation Rate (ESR) help detect underlying inflammation. Elevated CRP is associated with a higher risk of cardiovascular disease.[74,75]
- **Lipid Profile**
  includes total cholesterol, triglycerides, LDL, and HDL. According to the diagnostic criteria for metabolic syndrome, concern arises when:
  - Triglycerides > 1.7 mmol/L

- o HDL < 1.0 mmol/L for men, < 1.29 mmol/L for women

  I also pay close attention to the **triglyceride-to-HDL ratio**, aiming for less than 1.5.
- **Fasting Blood Glucose**

  ideally under 5.5 mmol/L. Readings above this suggest insulin resistance or risk of diabetes.
- **HbA1c** (Haemoglobin A1c)
  - o < 5.6%: Ideal
  - o 5.7–6.4%: Pre-diabetes
  - o ≥ 6.5%: Diagnostic of diabetes
- **Fasting Insulin**

  Though not always routinely tested, I find it very helpful. Ideal fasting insulin is around 5 mIU/L.
- **Vitamin D**

  It is essential not just for bone health but also for immunity, inflammation control, brain function, and cardiovascular protection:
  - o Lab normal: > 50 nmol/L
  - o Optimal: > 75, ideally over 100 nmol/L

    Deficiency is linked to osteoporosis, heart disease, autoimmune conditions, infections, and some cancers.
- **Iron Studies**

  Particularly **serum ferritin**, which reflects iron stores. I aim for a ferritin level of at least 30–50 ng/mL. Low levels can be due to inadequate red meat intake or other factors.

- **Vitamin B12**
  Found only in animal products, so vegetarians and vegans are at higher risk of deficiency:
    o Lab normal: > 200 pmol/L
    o Optimal: > 500 pmol/L for better energy and neurological health.

Coronary Artery Calcium (CAC) Score

The **CAC score** is a specialised CT scan that measures calcium deposits in the coronary arteries. It's an excellent tool for assessing heart attack risk:

- **Score of 0**: No detectable calcium – very low risk of a cardiovascular event in the next 10 years.[76]
- **Score > 100**: Indicates higher risk, warranting more intensive lifestyle and medical interventions.

NB: If a CAC score is elevated, I will often refer to a cardiologist for further evaluation and to help personalise the care plan.

What About Medications

While I prescribe lifestyle medicine, I am also a doctor with over 20 years of experience in prescribing medications. I firmly believe that medications have their place in healthcare.

Having spent the past five years focused on lifestyle medicine, I've come to see that medications and lifestyle interventions should be viewed as complementary, not as opposing choices.

In the lifestyle space, there's often resistance to medications. While I absolutely prefer to see someone thrive without them, there are situations where health can be further optimised through a thoughtful combination of both medication and lifestyle changes.

In this chapter, I'll discuss several groups of medications that are either controversial or particularly relevant when aiming to improve health holistically. I encourage readers to consult a medical professional before adjusting or discontinuing medications.

Medications That May Be Reviewed Alongside Lifestyle Changes

Statins (Cholesterol-lowering medications)
are commonly prescribed for cardiovascular risk prevention and cholesterol management but may be overprescribed in some cases. The traditional focus on total cholesterol alone is outdated. I encourage a personalised approach that includes assessing overall cardiovascular risk using tools like the *Multi-Ethnic Study of Atherosclerosis (MESA) Risk Score and Coronary Age Calculator*. These help patients make informed decisions about whether statin therapy is right for them.

Blood Pressure Medications

(e.g. ACE inhibitors, ARBs, calcium channel blockers, beta-blockers, diuretics). These medications help lower blood pressure and reduce the risk of cardiovascular disease. However, lifestyle changes – such as improved diet, exercise, stress management, and weight loss – can often improve blood pressure and reduce the need for medication. Always consult your doctor before making any changes and monitor your blood pressure regularly.

Diabetes Medications (including Metformin)

Metformin is often used to improve insulin resistance and blood glucose control. It can be helpful, especially in the early stages of insulin resistance or type 2 diabetes. However, with dietary changes such as a low-carbohydrate approach, some diabetes medications – especially insulin, sulfonylureas, and SGLT2 inhibitors – may need to be reduced or discontinued to avoid dangerously low blood sugar levels. This must be done under medical supervision.

Proton Pump Inhibitors (PPIs)

PPIs are used to treat Gastro-Oesophageal Reflux Disease (GORD) or GERD. Reflux is often linked to dietary and lifestyle factors. Many people experience improvement through reducing carbohydrate intake, time-restricted eating, weight loss, and stress reduction, making medication reduction possible with guidance from a healthcare professional.

Other Medications That May Be Reduced with Lifestyle Change

With improvements in diet, exercise, stress management, and sleep, some people may be able to reduce:

- Sleep medications
- Pain medications
- Antidepressants or anti-anxiety medications
- Asthma medications

NB: This is not an exhaustive list; always consult your doctor before making any changes.

Menopausal Hormone Therapy (MHT)

While lifestyle changes can support hormonal balance, many women benefit from MHT to manage menopausal symptoms. When symptoms are well controlled, women often feel more capable of engaging in lifestyle change.

After the decline in MHT use following the *Women's Health Initiative,* updated research and the use of body-identical hormones have brought renewed confidence in its safety and benefits for many women, when prescribed thoughtfully.

Supplements

While some people may have deficiencies in their diet, especially when beginning lifestyle changes, supplements can be useful. Common deficiencies include vitamin D, iron, B12, iodine, zinc, and magnesium. In certain cases, targeted supplementation can support metabolic health and help restore balance.

That said, my primary focus remains on getting nutrients from real, whole foods and natural sources like sunlight. One supplement I often recommend is magnesium, especially taken at night. It's a mineral that many are low in due to depleted soil quality, and it can be particularly helpful for those under stress or with active lifestyles.

Next-Level Lifestyle Habits

If you've already built a strong foundation in the six pillars of lifestyle medicine – nutrition, exercise, sleep, stress management, community, and managing addictions – and you're eager to explore further, this section is for you. Here, I share a few additional tools and strategies that may enhance your health and well-being even more.

Sauna

I recently invested in an affordable infrared sauna. Last year, I struggled with persistent neck pain that lasted for several months. Despite seeing a physiotherapist and receiving multiple massage treatments, the discomfort lingered. Whether it was a coincidence or not, after a few weeks of regular sauna use, my neck pain completely resolved.

Sauna use offers a wide range of potential health benefits:[77]

- **Improved circulation and cardiovascular health**: The heat elevates heart rate and increases blood flow, supporting overall heart function.
- **Enhanced detoxification**: Sweating aids in the elimination of toxins from the body.
- **Relief of muscle and joint pain**: Sauna heat can ease chronic pain, arthritis, and post-exercise soreness.
- **Nervous system support**: The relaxing warmth activates the parasympathetic nervous system. Combined with mindfulness or meditation, it can significantly reduce stress.
- **Healthier skin**: Improved circulation and sweating may enhance skin tone, reduce acne, and promote a clearer complexion.
- **Metabolic support**: Some studies suggest that regular sauna use may improve insulin sensitivity, support weight management, and lower the risk of metabolic syndrome.

Cold Exposure

A couple of months before writing this book, I finally tried an ice bath. I had seen some friends regularly doing them, but it took me a few years to build up the courage. I signed up for a weekend workshop that included a 40-minute breathwork session, followed by an ice bath experience.

I had already made up my mind to give it a go, so when it was my turn, I didn't overthink it. I jumped in and, to my surprise, it wasn't as hard as I imagined. I stayed in for two minutes, got out, and felt exhilarated.

After that experience, I started experimenting at home by filling up my bathtub and adding frozen water bottles to cool it down. Cold exposure has many benefits – it boosts circulation, reduces inflammation, supports mental clarity, and enhances immune function. It also stimulates the release of dopamine and adrenaline, which can improve mood, alertness, and focus. Studies suggest cold exposure may increase brown fat, a metabolically active fat that helps burn energy and regulate body temperature and reduce white fat.[78]

Getting into a cold bath takes courage, but regular practice builds both tolerance and resilience. I've happily done ice baths through summer – whether this habit continues into Melbourne's winter remains to be seen!

Grounding/Earthing

I have also discovered the benefits of grounding. I started incorporating five to 10 minutes of grounding this summer after my walks or runs. I would take off my shoes at the end of the street after a run to walk on the grass or take breaks to soak up the sun and enjoy the feeling of my feet connecting with the earth. I hope to continue this practice in winter, even when it gets colder.

Grounding, also known as earthing, involves direct physical contact with the earth, such as walking barefoot on grass, soil, or sand, or even hugging a tree.

Grounding works by reconnecting the human body with the Earth's natural electric charge. When you make direct contact with the earth, free electrons flow from the ground into your body, helping to discharge any excess charge.

Modern lifestyles – marked by rubber-soled shoes and predominantly indoor living – tend to insulate us from the Earth's natural electrical charge. However, studies have shown that grounding can offer a range of health benefits. These include reduced stress, improved sleep quality, decreased daytime sleepiness, and enhanced cardiovascular health through better circulation.

Grounding also helps balance the autonomic nervous system, supports circadian rhythm regulation, and contributes to both physical and emotional well-being. Emerging evidence even suggests that it may reduce inflammation, promote wound healing, and support faster muscle recovery after exercise.[79,80]

Becoming Aware of the Chemicals in Your Environment

It can feel overwhelming how much we need to change, but the key is noticing and learning, taking small steps at a time. While the full list of chemicals we encounter is beyond the scope of this book, this short, non-exhaustive list can encourage you to continue learning.

- **Plastics**: Found in plastic containers, food packaging, and water bottles. These may contain chemicals that leach into food and drinks, especially when heated.[81]
- **Personal care products**: Many cosmetics, lotions, shampoos, and deodorants contain parabens, which may disrupt the endocrine system and affect hormonal balance.[82]
- **Non-stick cookware**: Items like non-stick pans may contain per fluorinated chemicals (PFCs) that can leach into food when heated, particularly at high temperatures.
- **Contaminated water**: Heavy metals, pesticides, and fertilisers can contaminate water, seafood, and crops, contributing to the accumulation of harmful substances in the body.[83]

Some of these chemicals are classified as probable carcinogens, meaning long-term exposure may increase the risk of certain cancers.[84] Others can mimic oestrogen and disrupt hormonal balance, potentially increasing the risk of metabolic diseases such as obesity, insulin resistance, and type 2 diabetes.

Top 10 Tips for Lifestyle Success

1. Identify Your Why

Reflect on the reason you bought and are reading this book.

Is it because you want to lose weight? Be healthier, live longer, and have more energy? Do you want to be able to play with your grandchildren? Stay in your own home and avoid moving into a nursing home? Avoid becoming frail and needing a walking frame in older age? Prevent dementia and keep a sharp mind as you age? Do you have children overseas and want to continue travelling by air to visit them in later life? Do you want to enjoy retirement and have the energy to travel the world and explore without limits?

It may be helpful to write your reason down.

2. Set Clear and Achievable Goals

Break down larger goals into smaller ones. The SMART method can be useful. For example, if your goal is weight loss:

'I will lose 4g in the next eight weeks by walking 30 minutes, five days a week, and following a low-carb lifestyle.'

Let's be SMART:

- **Specific**: Lose 4kg with walking and a low-carb way of eating
- **Measurable**: 4kg weight loss
- **Achievable**: Ensure it's realistic in the timeframe
- **Relevant**: Supports your health and weight loss goals
- **Time-bound**: Eight weeks

3. Start Small, Build One Habit at a Time

Begin with small, achievable changes. Don't try to change everything at once – it can be overwhelming. Focus on one change at a time.

For example, start by switching your breakfast from cereal to eggs. Some patients I work with adopt a new habit with each visit. One might reduce sugar intake first, then lower carbohydrate intake at the next visit, exercise, and later begin breathwork. One step at a time.

It's helpful to build a consistent routine. You could schedule habits in your diary. Use a habit tracker to tick off healthy behaviours each day. Maybe Sunday afternoon becomes your meal prep day. Your weekly routine might look like this: Monday strength training, Tuesday running, Wednesday strength, Thursday running, and so on. Once habits are embedded, they become second nature and don't require extra planning.

4. The K.E.Y. is to Keep Educating Yourself

Empower yourself by continuing to learn – you need to take charge of your own health. Learn about the benefits of the changes you are making.

Each section of this book includes further learning suggestions and people you can follow. Read more books. Take courses. Follow experts on social media. Deepen your understanding of nutrition, exercise, and stress management. Try to understand the science behind it all. If it doesn't make sense at first, that's okay – learning takes time. One of my professors in medical school used to say, *"The secret to success is constant repetition."*

5. Life Begins at the End of Your Comfort Zone

Starting something new is hard and awkward. It takes courage to build new habits. Doing hard things strengthens resilience, and discomfort is where growth happens. Whether you're stretching your limits, changing your diet, or trying breathwork, you're building new pathways in your brain and body.

Growth doesn't happen in a comfort zone.

Building hardiness makes you stronger physically, mentally, psychologically, and spiritually. As you conquer small challenges, your confidence grows, and when bigger stressors come your way, you're better equipped to handle them and bounce back faster.

Doing hard things is not punishment. It's training. It's a gift to your future self.

6. Track Progress and Reflect
Journaling can be a powerful tool to track how you feel and your progress over time.

Regular GP visits and blood tests every three months can help monitor your metabolic health.

You can also use a journal, an app, or a calendar to track habits, mood, and outcomes. This builds self-awareness and keeps motivation high.

7. Check in With Your Mind – Chaos or Calm
Ask yourself: Is this action helping your mind? For example, if you eat a piece of cake, ask yourself: 'Will this create chaos or calm in my mind?'

If it leaves you feeling guilty or leads to self-blame, it may not be worth it. But if the same piece of cake is at your grandchild's birthday party, and you feel joy in participating and connection in being present, and you return to healthy eating the next meal, it may create calm, not chaos. Let your mind be your guide.

8. Celebrate Wins Big and Small
Celebrate both big and small achievements.

If you've successfully replaced *Diet Coke* with soda water – celebrate! If you've lost 2kg a month but stalled over the Christmas holidays, celebrate that you maintained your weight.

9. Seek Support – It's Strong to Ask for Help

It's okay to ask for help. In fact, it's a strength. Helping people with lifestyle changes is what I do – and I love doing it.

The internet is filled with conflicting information, and you don't always know what advice is suitable for your situation. Sometimes all it takes is a consultation to point you in the right direction.

If you've fallen off track due to a stressful time, reach out. I would be absolutely delighted to receive a message or email asking for help to get back on track. Most health professionals feel the same – we're here to support you.

10. Enjoy the Journey

Lifestyle changes are rewarding. It's time to put yourself first – not your partner, not your kids, not your parents. If you don't care for yourself, you can't care for others.

This isn't selfish – it's <u>self-compassion</u>.

The journey becomes enjoyable when you begin to discover what works for you. You'll feel better, achieve your goals, improve your blood markers, lose weight, boost your energy, and reduce bloating. I've even seen women with polycystic ovarian syndrome (PCOS) who have struggled with infertility go on to conceive naturally after embracing a low-carb lifestyle.

That is the power of change.

AFTERWORD

———————— ◆ ◇ ◆ ————————

*P*rescribing Lifestyle: A Doctor's Prescription for Lasting Weight Loss and Vibrant Health is not just a book – it's my mission.

As a doctor with over 20 years of experience, I've seen the burden of chronic disease up close. But in the last five years, I've witnessed something extraordinary: when patients embrace lifestyle change, they transform their health, energy, and well-being.

Many have lost weight and kept it off. Others have reversed chronic conditions and reduced or stopped medications. Some with mental health conditions have had dramatic improvement. Most importantly, they've felt better – more vibrant, more alive.

My mission is to spread the message that lasting weight loss and vibrant health don't come from quick fixes, but from consistent, meaningful changes.

I invite you to take ownership of your health. Explore new ways of living that go beyond diets and fads. Build habits that support a thriving, resilient version of you.

If this book has sparked something in you – a fresh insight, a new habit, a sense of possibility – please share it. Tell a friend, a family member, or a colleague who might benefit. You never know whose life you might change.

Together, we can create a ripple effect of empowered individuals, healthy choices, and communities that support one another in thriving.

Let this be your invitation to take the first step – and to invite others to walk alongside you on the journey to lasting health and vitality.

ABOUT THE AUTHOR

—————————— ◆◇◆ ——————————

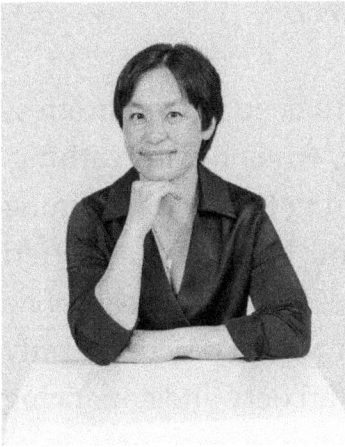

Dr Avi Charlton is a General Practitioner who graduated from the *University of Melbourne* in 2000. She has been practising family medicine for over 20 years, treating anything that comes through the door. In recent years, she developed a special interest in lifestyle medicine, focusing on nutrition, exercise, sleep, stress management, breathing, and connecting with the community.

Born in Hong Kong and of Chinese heritage, Dr Charlton is married to an Australian man. Together, they have two teenage boys, ages 13 and 16.

She founded *Melbourne Low Carb Clinic* in 2022 with the aim of taking a holistic approach to providing health care and nutritional information. She discusses eating a real-food diet and other lifestyle pillars to optimise her patients' health. She has helped improve chronic conditions such as type 2 diabetes, obesity, polycystic ovarian syndrome, mental health conditions, etc.

She is affiliated with *Low Carb Down Under, Diet Doctor* and is an accredited Metabolic Health Practitioner with the *Society of Metabolic Health Practitioners* (SMHP) and *Australasian Metabolic Health Society.*

Her work in lifestyle also sparked a deep interest in stress management and, in particular, functional breathing. She completed Functional Breathing Instructor Training with *The Oxygen Advantage* and became a certified breathwork facilitator through the *Breathless Academy.* She now integrates breathwork into medical practice, firmly believing in its role in managing anxiety and enhancing overall well-being.

Dr Charlton founded *Breathe in Health,* a platform dedicated to promoting functional breathing and breathwork practices. Through this, she offers one-on-one breathing coaching, breathwork workshops, group sessions, and retreats to help individuals improve their health through their breath.

Outside her clinical role, Dr Charlton is a passionate runner. She has completed two full marathons and walked the 100km *Oxfam* challenge. She continues to walk, run, and strength train to maintain physical health.

In 2024, Dr Charlton launched a podcast, *Prescribing Lifestyle*, which is approaching 100 episodes to date. Through conversations with fellow health professionals, colleagues, and inspiring individuals, the podcast explores practical strategies for living better through lifestyle medicine.

Dr Charlton is committed to helping spread the word about integrating nutrition, breathing, and holistic lifestyle strategies to live longer, healthier lives.

ACKNOWLEDGEMENTS

$\bullet \diamond \bullet$

Writing *Prescribing Lifestyle* has been a journey of reflection, learning, and deep gratitude.

To my patients, thank you for trusting me with your stories, struggles and triumphs. You've taught me more than any textbook ever could.

To my husband and two sons, thank you for your love, patience, and support. You made everything possible. You keep me grounded and remind me why this work matters.

To my colleagues and friends in the low-carb and lifestyle medicine community – Dr Peter Brukner, Carla Veith-Carter, Tracey McBeath, Gillian Harvey, Dr Lucy Burns, and many more – your passion, collaboration, and friendship have enriched this journey beyond words. Thank you.

To the members of *Low Carb Melbourne* and the *Melbourne Low Carb Clinic Free community* – thank you for showing up, sharing openly, and supporting one another so generously. You've built a space of encouragement and real transformation. And to the *Low Carb Pro* members, your commitment and strength continue to inspire me during our fortnightly *Zoom* sessions.

And finally, to the *Prescribing Lifestyle* podcast listeners – your enthusiasm and feedback across nearly 100 episodes have helped shape this message and bring it to life. Thank you.

This book is for you all.

3 WAYS TO WORK WITH ME

————————— ◆◇◆ —————————

1. Book a Personal Consultation

Join me for a comprehensive one-on-one consultation to explore your health goals, medical history, and current lifestyle. We'll create a tailored nutrition and lifestyle plan to support your well-being and long-term health.

2. Follow Me Online and Tune in to the Podcast

Stay connected via social media and my *Prescribing Lifestyle* podcast, where I share practical tips, expert insights, and the latest science on nutrition, breathwork, mental health, and more. As research evolves, so will the information I provide – always rooted in evidence and real-life experience.

3. Invite Me to Speak

I'm passionate about sharing the power of healthy living. If you're an employer or an event organiser, inviting me to speak to your team could inspire positive lifestyle changes, improve health literacy, and support productivity and well-being in the workplace.

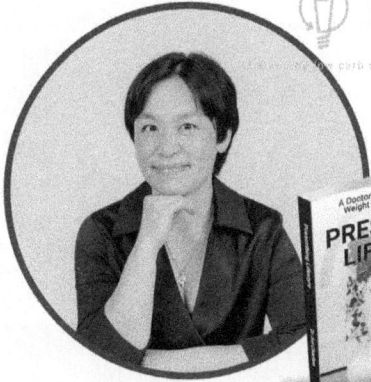

Dr Avi Charlton

*Lifestyle General Practitioner, Speaker,
Author, Podcast Host, Mum of 2 boys*

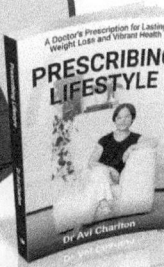

A Doctor's Prescription for Lasting
Weight Loss and Vibrant Health

**PRESCRIBING
LIFESTYLE**

Dr Avi Charlton

✉ avi.charlton@mlcclinic.com.au

🌐 www.mlcclinic.com.au

🎙 Prescribing Lifestyle Podcast

f @dr charlton lifestyle GP ⬡ @dr charlton lifestyle GP in @Avi Charlton

About Avi

Dr. Charlton is the founder of the Melbourne Low Carb Clinic, a specialised GP clinic dedicated to promoting healthy nutrition and lifestyle. Since its inception in October 2022, the clinic has been providing comprehensive consultations lasting up to 45 minutes. In addition to medical consultations, Dr. Charlton offers online courses and membership programs to educate and support members on their journey toward better health.

With over 20 years of experience as a family doctor, Dr. Charlton has developed a keen interest in nutrition, obesity treatment, metabolic syndrome, and functional breathing. She has pursued extensive education in these areas and has successfully treated numerous patients for weight management. Her expertise in the low carbohydrate approach has helped patients lose weight, improve their nutrition, and even reverse conditions such as metabolic syndrome and diabetes.

Dr. Charlton not only advocates for low carb nutrition but also practices it herself. In her leisure time, she has embraced endurance running and strength training, completing two full marathons in the last three years while adhering to a low carbohydrate diet.

In addition to her clinical work, Dr. Charlton has launched her podcast and has been a guest on various other podcasts, sharing her knowledge and experience in nutrition, lifestyle medicine, and functional breathing.

Speaking Topics

- The Foundations of Optimal Living: How to Master the Six Pillars of Lifestyle for Better Health
- How to Lose Weight Without Feeling Hungry: A Science-Backed Approach to Sustainable Health
- Breathe Your Way to Calm: Managing Stress and Anxiety with the Power of Breathing

FEATURED IN:

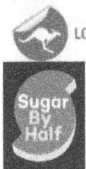

LOW CARB DOWN UNDER

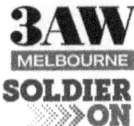

3AW MELBOURNE

Sugar By Half

SOLDIER ON

REJUVENATE
HEALTH & FITNESS RETREATS

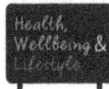

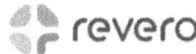

Health, Wellbeing & Lifestyle

revero

InsightTimer

REAL LIFE MEDICINE

Australian Weight Loss Summit

REFERENCES

◆◇◆

Introduction

1 World Health Organization. (n.d.). Obesity and overweight. Retrieved [Date], from https://www.who.int/news-room/fact-sheets/detail/obesity-and-overweight

2 Obesity Evidence Hub https://www.obesityevidencehub.org.au/collections/trends/adults-global

3 https://www.aihw.gov.au/reports/overweight-obesity/overweight-and-obesity/contents/

4 https://www.who.int/news/item/01-03-2024-one-in-eight-people-are-now-living-with-obesity

5 NCD Risk Factor Collaboration (NCD-RisC). (2024). Worldwide trends in underweight and obesity from 1990 to 2022: A pooled analysis of 3,663 population-representative studies with 222 million children, adolescents, and adults. The Lancet, 403(10431), 1027–1050. https://doi.org/10.1016/S0140-6736(23)02750-2

6 NCD Risk Factor Collaboration (NCD-RisC). (2024). Worldwide trends in diabetes prevalence and treatment from 1990 to 2022: A pooled analysis of 1,108 population-representative

studies with 141 million participants. The Lancet, 404(10683), 2077–2093. https://doi.org/10.1016/S0140-6736(24)02317-

[7] Australian Institute of Health and Welfare (AIHW). (2024). Chronic conditions. Retrieved from https://www.aihw.gov.au/reports/australias-health/chronic-conditions

[8] Al Jazeera. (2021, October 17). Australia's Melbourne set to end world's longest lockdowns. https://www.aljazeera.com/news/2021/10/17/australias-melbourne-set-to-end-worlds-longest-lockdowns

[9] Diabetes deaths: Australian Institute of Health and Welfare (AIHW). (2024). Diabetes: Australian facts. Retrieved from https://www.aihw.gov.au/reports/diabetes/diabetes/contents/impact-of-diabetes/diabetes-deaths

[10] COVID-19 deaths: Australian Bureau of Statistics (ABS). (2023). Causes of Death, Australia, 2022. Retrieved from https://www.abs.gov.au/statistics/health/causes-death/causes-death-australia/2022

[11] Australian Bureau of Statistics. (2024, November 8). Life expectancy, 2021–2023. https://www.abs.gov.au/statistics/people/population/life-expectancy/latest-release

[12] Australian Institute of Health and Welfare. (2023). Australian Burden of Disease Study 2023. https://www.aihw.gov.au/reports/burden-of-disease/australian-burden-of-disease-study-2023

Chapter 2

[13] https://isupportgary.com/ by Belinda Fettke

[14] The Global Influence of the Seventh-Day Adventist Church on Diet, Religions 2018, 9(9), 251; https://doi.org/10.3390/rel9090251

[15] Yudkin, John. Pure, White and Deadly: How Sugar Is Killing Us and What We Can Do to Stop It. London: Penguin Books, 2012.

[16] Keys A, Menotti A, Aravanis C, Blackburn H, Djordevic BS, Buzina R, Dontas AS, Fidanza F, Karvonen MJ, Kimura N, et al. The seven countries study: 2,289 deaths in 15 years. Prev Med. 1984 Mar;13(2):141-54. doi: 10.1016/0091-7435(84)90047-1. PMID: 6739443.

[17] U.S. Senate Select Committee on Nutrition and Human Needs. Dietary Goals for the United States. 2nd ed. Washington, DC: U.S. Government Printing Office, 1977.

[18] National Health and Medical Research Council. (2013). Australian Dietary Guidelines (1st ed.). Canberra: National Health and Medical Research Council. https://www.nhmrc. gov.au/about-us/publications/australian-dietary-guidelines

[19] Oxford Magazine. (2024, May 8). British daily meat consumption drops by 17% over a decade, Oxford study finds. https://theoxfordmagazine.com/news/british-daily-meat-consumption-drops-by-17-over-a-decade-oxford-study-finds/

Chapter 3

[20] de Souza, R. J., Mente, A., Maroleanu, A., Cozma, A. I., Ha, V., Kishibe, T., Uleryk, E., Budylowski, P., Schünemann, H. J., Beyene, J., & Anand, S. S. (2020). Intake of saturated and trans unsaturated fatty acids and risk of all-cause mortality, cardiovascular disease, and type 2 diabetes: Systematic review and meta-analysis of observational studies. Journal of the American College of Cardiology, 76(16), 2007–2022. https://doi.org/10.1016/j.jacc.2020.05.077

[21] Zhu, XF., Hu, YQ., Dai, ZC. et al. Associations between trans fatty acids and systemic immune-inflammation index: a

cross-sectional study. *Lipids Health Dis* **23**, 122 (2024). https://doi.org/10.1186/s12944-024-02109-w

Chapter 4

[22] Carson, J. A. S., Lichtenstein, A. H., Anderson, C. A. M., Appel, L. J., Kris-Etherton, P. M., Meyer, K. A., ... & Wylie-Rosett, J. (2020). Dietary cholesterol and cardiovascular risk: A science advisory from the American Heart Association. Circulation, 141(3), e39–e53. https://doi.org/10.1161/CIR.0000000000000743

[23] Ginsberg, H. N., Packard, C. J., Chapman, M. J., et al. (2021). Triglyceride-rich lipoproteins and their remnants: metabolic insights, role in atherosclerotic cardiovascular disease, and emerging therapeutic strategies—a consensus statement from the European Atherosclerosis Society. European Heart Journal, 42(47), 4791–4806. https://doi.org/10.1093/eurheartj/ehab551

[24] Araújo, J., Cai, J., Stevens, J., & Preiss, D. (2019). Prevalence of optimal metabolic health in American adults: National Health and Nutrition Examination Survey 2009–2016. Metabolic Syndrome and Related Disorders, 17(1), 46–52. https://doi.org/10.1089/met.2018.0105 PMID: 30484738

[25] Haridas B, Testino A, Kossoff EH. Ketogenic diet therapy for the treatment of pediatric epilepsy. Epileptic Disord. 2025 Apr;27(2):144-155. doi: 10.1002/epd2.20320. Epub 2024 Dec 12. PMID: 39665749; PMCID: PMC12065128.

[26] Brukner, P. (2018). A fat lot of good. Pan Macmillan Australia.

[27] Wang, X., Bao, W., Liu, J., Ouyang, Y. Y., Wang, D., Rong, S., ... & Liu, L. (2013). Inflammatory markers and risk of type 2 diabetes: A systematic review and meta-analysis. Diabetes Care, 36(1), 166–175. https://doi.org/10.2337/dc12-0702

[28] Qin, P., Ho, F.K., Celis-Morales, C.A. et al. Association between systemic inflammation biomarkers and incident cardiovascular disease in 423,701 individuals: evidence from the UK biobank cohort. Cardiovasc Diabetol 24, 162 (2025). https://doi.org/10.1186/s12933-025-02721-9

[29] Danesh, J., et al. (2000). Low grade inflammation and coronary heart disease: prospective study and updated meta-analyses. BMJ, 321(7255), 199–204. https://doi.org/10.1136/bmj.321.7255.199

[30] Gkrinia, E. M. M., & Belančić, A. (2025). The Mechanisms of Chronic Inflammation in Obesity and Potential Therapeutic Strategies: A Narrative Review. Current Issues in Molecular Biology, 47(5), 357. https://doi.org/10.3390/cimb47050357

[31] Dahiya, M., Yadav, M., Goyal, C. et al. Insulin resistance in Alzheimer's disease: signalling mechanisms and therapeutics strategies. *Inflammopharmacol* **33**, 1817–1831 (2025). https://doi.org/10.1007/s10787-025-01704-2

[32] Mazza, M. G., Lucchi, S., Tringali, A. G. M., Rossetti, A., Botti, R. E., & Clerici, M. (2024). Inflammatory biomarkers and depression: A systematic review. *Neuroscience & Biobehavioral Reviews*, 159, 105528. https://doi.org/10.1016/j.neubiorev.2024.105528

[33] Coussens, L., Werb, Z. Inflammation and cancer. Nature 420, 860–867 (2002). https://doi.org/10.1038/nature01322

Chapter 6

[34] Wang, Z., Wang, J. The effects of high-intensity interval training versus moderate-intensity continuous training on athletes' aerobic endurance performance parameters. Eur J Appl Physiol 124, 2235–2249 (2024). https://doi.org/10.1007/s00421-024-05532-0

[35] Batacan Jr, R. B., Duncan, M. J., Dalbo, V. J., Tucker, P. S., & Fenning, A. S. (2017). Effects of high-intensity interval training on cardiometabolic health: A systematic review and meta-analysis of intervention studies. British Journal of Sports Medicine, 51(6), 494–503. https://doi.org/10.1136/bjsports-2015-095841

[36] Mosti MP, Kaehler N, Stunes AK, Hoff J, Syversen U. Maximal strength training in postmenopausal women with osteoporosis or osteopenia. J Strength Cond Res. 2013 Oct;27(10):2879-86. doi: 10.1519/JSC.0b013e318280d4e2. PMID: 23287836.

[37] Lu L, Mao L, Feng Y, Ainsworth BE, Liu Y, Chen N. Effects of different exercise training modes on muscle strength and physical performance in older people with sarcopenia: a systematic review and meta-analysis. BMC Geriatr. 2021 Dec 15;21(1):708. doi: 10.1186/s12877-021-02642-8. PMID: 34911483; PMCID: PMC8672633.

[38] Noetel M, Sanders T, Gallardo-Gómez D, Taylor P, Del Pozo Cruz B, van den Hoek D, Smith JJ, Mahoney J, Spathis J, Moresi M, Pagano R, Pagano L, Vasconcellos R, Arnott H, Varley B, Parker P, Biddle S, Lonsdale C. Effect of exercise for depression: systematic review and network meta-analysis of randomised controlled trials. BMJ. 2024 Feb 14;384: e075847. doi: 10.1136/bmj-2023-075847. Erratum in: BMJ. 2024 May 28;385: q1024. doi: 10.1136/bmj. q1024. PMID: 38355154; PMCID: PMC10870815.

[39] Bocchicchio, B. (n.d.). SMaRT Program: Slow MAximum Response Training.

[40] Cheng AJ, Jude B, Lanner JT. Intramuscular mechanisms of overtraining. Redox Biol. 2020 Aug; 35:101480. doi: 10.1016/j.redox.2020.101480. Epub 2020 Feb 26. PMID: 32179050; PMCID: PMC7284919.

Chapter 8

[41] Watson, N. F., Martin, J. L., Wise, M. S., Carden, K. A., & Curhan, G. C. (2015). Joint consensus statement of the American Academy of Sleep Medicine and Sleep Research Society on the recommended amount of sleep for a healthy adult: Methodology and discussion. Journal of Clinical Sleep Medicine, 11(8), 931–952. https://doi.org/10.5664/jcsm.4950

[42] American Academy of Sleep Medicine. (n.d.). Recommended amount of sleep for a healthy adult: A consensus statement. Retrieved [Date], from https://aasm.org/recommended-amount-of-sleep/

[43] Sleep Foundation. (n.d.). Sleep statistics. Retrieved [Date], from https://www.sleepfoundation.org/how-sleep-works/how-much-sleep-do-we-really-need

[44] HealthMatch. (n.d.). Too many of us are sleep deprived and It's become a crisis. Retrieved [Date], from https://healthmatch.io/blog/sleep-deprivation-crisis

Chapter 9

[45] Aulsebrook AE, Jones TM, Mulder RA, Lesku JA. Impacts of artificial light at night on sleep: A review and prospectus. J Exp Zool A Ecol Integr Physiol. 2018 Oct;329(8-9):409-418. doi: 10.1002/jez.2189. Epub 2018 Jun 4. PMID: 29869374.

[46] Cho Y, Ryu SH, Lee BR, Kim KH, Lee E, Choi J. Effects of artificial light at night on human health: A literature review of observational and experimental studies applied to exposure assessment. Chronobiol Int. 2015;32(9):1294-310. doi: 10.3109/07420528.2015.1073158. Epub 2015 Sep 16. PMID: 26375320.

[47] Pauley SM. Lighting for the human circadian clock: recent research indicates that lighting has become a public health

issue. Med Hypotheses. 2004;63(4):588-96. doi: 10.1016/j. mehy.2004.03.020. PMID: 15325001.

[48] Depner CM, Stothard ER, Wright KP Jr. Metabolic consequences of sleep and circadian disorders. Curr Diab Rep. 2014 Jul;14(7):507. doi: 10.1007/s11892-014-0507-z. PMID: 24816752; PMCID: PMC4308960.

Chapter 10

[49] Lupien SJ, Juster RP, Raymond C, Marin MF. The effects of chronic stress on the human brain: From neurotoxicity, to vulnerability, to opportunity. Front Neuroendocrinol. 2018 Apr;49:91-105. doi: 10.1016/j.yfrne.2018.02.001. Epub 2018 Feb 5. PMID: 29421159.

[50] Noushad S, Ahmed S, Ansari B, Mustafa UH, Saleem Y, Hazrat H. Physiological biomarkers of chronic stress: A systematic review. Int J Health Sci (Qassim). 2021 Sep-Oct;15(5):46-59. PMID: 34548863; PMCID: PMC8434839.

[51] Resmini E, Santos A, Webb SM. Cortisol Excess and the Brain. Front Horm Res. 2016;46:74-86. doi: 10.1159/000443868. Epub 2016 May 17. PMID: 27210466.

[52] Price RB, Duman R. Neuroplasticity in cognitive and psychological mechanisms of depression: an integrative model. Mol Psychiatry. 2020 Mar;25(3):530-543. doi: 10.1038/s41380-019-0615-x. Epub 2019 Dec 4. PMID: 31801966; PMCID: PMC7047599.

Chapter 11

[53] McKeown, P. (2015). The Oxygen Advantage: The Simple, Scientifically Proven Breathing Technique That Will Revolutionize Your Health and Fitness. HarperOne.

References

[54] Nestor, J. (2020). Breath: The New Science of a Lost Art. Riverhead Books.

[55] Zhao Z, Zheng L, Huang X, Li C, Liu J, Hu Y. Effects of mouth breathing on facial skeletal development in children: a systematic review and meta-analysis. BMC Oral Health. 2021 Mar 10;21(1):108. doi: 10.1186/s12903-021-01458-7. PMID: 33691678; PMCID: PMC7944632.

[56] Araújo BCL, de Magalhães Simões S, de Gois-Santos VT, Martins-Filho PRS. Association Between Mouth Breathing and Asthma: a Systematic Review and Meta-analysis. Curr Allergy Asthma Rep. 2020 May 19;20(7):24. doi: 10.1007/s11882-020-00921-9. PMID: 32430704.

[57] Newson TP, Elias A. Breathing pattern disorders (dysfunctional breathing) characteristics and outcomes of children and young people attending a secondary care respiratory clinic. Pediatr Pulmonol. 2020 Jul;55(7):1736-1744. doi: 10.1002/ppul.24791. Epub 2020 May 25. PMID: 32449843.

[58] Kalaskar R, Bhaje P, Kalaskar A, Faye A. Sleep Difficulties and Symptoms of Attention-deficit Hyperactivity Disorder in Children with Mouth Breathing. Int J Clin Pediatr Dent. 2021 Sep-Oct;14(5):604-609. doi: 10.5005/jp-journals-10005-1987. PMID: 34934269; PMCID: PMC8645617.

[59] Naik GS, Gaur GS, Pal GK. Effect of Modified Slow Breathing Exercise on Perceived Stress and Basal Cardiovascular Parameters. Int J Yoga. 2018 Jan-Apr;11(1):53-58. doi: 10.4103/ijoy.IJOY_41_16. PMID: 29343931; PMCID: PMC5769199.

[60] Giorgi F, Tedeschi R. Breathe better, live better: the science of slow breathing and heart rate variability. Acta Neurol Belg. 2025 Apr 19. doi: 10.1007/s13760-025-02789-w. Epub ahead of print. PMID: 40252198.

[61] Garg P, Mendiratta A, Banga A, Bucharles A, Victoria P, Kamaraj B, Qasba RK, Bansal V, Thimmapuram J, Pargament

R, Kashyap R. Effect of breathing exercises on blood pressure and heart rate: A systematic review and meta-analysis. Int J Cardiol Cardiovasc Risk Prev. 2023 Dec 27;20:200232. doi: 10.1016/j.ijcrp.2023.200232. PMID: 38179185; PMCID: PMC10765252.

[62] Obaya HE, Abdeen HA, Salem AA, Shehata MA, Aldhahi MI, Muka T, Marques-Sule E, Taha MM, Gaber M, Atef H. Effect of aerobic exercise, slow deep breathing and mindfulness meditation on cortisol and glucose levels in women with type 2 diabetes mellitus: a randomized controlled trial. Front Physiol. 2023 Jul 13;14:1186546. doi: 10.3389/fphys.2023.1186546. PMID: 37520826; PMCID: PMC10373883.

[63] Komase Y, Watanabe K, Hori D, Nozawa K, Hidaka Y, Iida M, Imamura K, Kawakami N. Effects of gratitude intervention on mental health and well-being among workers: A systematic review. J Occup Health. 2021 Jan;63(1):e12290. doi: 10.1002/1348-9585.12290. PMID: 34762326; PMCID: PMC8582291.

Chapter 12

[64] Lifestyle modification for the management of obesity. The Journal of the American Medical Association, 302(5), 593–595. https://doi.org/10.1001/jama.2009.1069

[65] Health coaching for chronic disease management: A systematic review. American Journal of Lifestyle Medicine, 6(3), 196-204. https://doi.org/10.1177/1559827612437769

[66] Health coaching and its impact on metabolic syndrome risk factors. Preventive Medicine, 71, 70–75. https://doi.org/10.1016/j.ypmed.2014.11.010

[67] A systematic review of the effectiveness of health coaching on physical activity outcomes. British Journal of Health Psychology, 24(3), 425-444. https://doi.org/10.1111/bjhp.12344

Chapter 13

[68] Felitti, V. J., Anda, R. F., Nordenberg, D., Williamson, D. F., Spitz, A. M., Edwards, V., ... & Marks, J. S. (1998).Relationship of childhood abuse and household dysfunction to many of the leading causes of death in adults: The Adverse Childhood Experiences (ACE) Study. *American Journal of Preventive Medicine*, 14(4), 245–258. https://doi.org/10.1016/S0749-3797(98)00017-8

[69] Hughes, K., Bellis, M. A., Hardcastle, K. A., Sethi, D., Butchart, A., Mikton, C., ... & Dunne, M. P. (2017). The effect of multiple adverse childhood experiences on health: a systematic review and meta-analysis. BMC Public Health, 17(1), 1–10. https://doi.org/10.1186/s12889-016-2906-3

[70] O'Brien CP. The CAGE Questionnaire for Detection of Alcoholism. JAMA. 2008;300(17):2054–2056. doi:10.1001/jama.2008.570

[71] Hoffmann, N. G., Hunt, D. E., Rhodes, W. M., & Riley, K. J. (2003). UNCOPE: A Brief Substance Dependence Screen for Use with Arrestees. Journal of Drug Issues, 33(1), 29-44. https://doi.org/10.1177/002204260303300102 (Original work published 2003)

[72] Unwin J, Delon C, Giæver H, Kennedy C, Painschab M, Sandin F, Poulsen CS, Wiss DA. Low carbohydrate and psychoeducational programs show promise for the treatment of ultra-processed food addiction. Front Psychiatry. 2022 Sep 28;13:1005523. doi: 10.3389/fpsyt.2022.1005523. PMID: 36245868; PMCID: PMC9554504.

[73] Carmen M, Safer DL, Saslow LR, Kalayjian T, Mason AE, Westman EC, Sethi S. Treating binge eating and food addiction symptoms with low-carbohydrate Ketogenic diets: a case series. J Eat Disord. 2020 Jan 29;8:2. doi: 10.1186/s40337-020-0278-7. Erratum in: J Eat Disord. 2023 Sep 29;11(1):171.

doi: 10.1186/s40337-023-00881-1. PMID: 32010444; PMCID: PMC6988301.

Going Forward

[74] C-reactive protein and other markers of inflammation in the prediction of cardiovascular disease in women. N Engl J Med. 2000 Mar 23;342(12):836-43

[75] Inflammatory cytokines and risk of coronary heart disease: new prospective study and updated meta-analysis. Eur Heart J. 2014 Dec 1;35(9):578-89.

[76] Sheppard JP, Lakshmanan S, Lichtenstein SJ, Budoff MJ, Roy SK. Age and the power of zero CAC in cardiac risk assessment: overview of the literature and a cautionary case. Br J Cardiol. 2022 Jul 19;29(3):23. doi: 10.5837/bjc.2022.023. PMID: 36873724; PMCID: PMC9982666.

[77] Laukkanen JA, Kunutsor SK. The multifaceted benefits of passive heat therapies for extending the health span: A comprehensive review with a focus on Finnish sauna. Temperature (Austin). 2024 Feb 25;11(1):27-51. doi: 10.1080/23328940.2023.2300623. PMID: 38577299; PMCID: PMC10989710.

[78] Huttunen, P., Rintamäki, H., & Hirvonen, J. (2018). Capacity for nonshivering thermogenesis and brown adipose tissue in healthy adults. American Journal of Physiology-Regulatory, Integrative and Comparative Physiology, 314(3), R287–R295. https://doi.org/10.1152/ajpregu.00115.2017

[79] Oschman JL, Chevalier G, Brown R. The effects of grounding (earthing) on inflammation, the immune response, wound healing, and prevention and treatment of chronic inflammatory and autoimmune diseases. J Inflamm Res. 2015 Mar 24;8:83-96. doi: 10.2147/JIR.S69656. PMID: 25848315; PMCID: PMC4378297.

References

[80] Sinatra ST, Sinatra DS, Sinatra SW, Chevalier G. Grounding - The universal anti-inflammatory remedy. Biomed J. 2023 Feb;46(1):11-16. doi: 10.1016/j.bj.2022.12.002. Epub 2022 Dec 15. PMID: 36528336; PMCID: PMC10105021.

[81] Donisi I, Colloca A, Anastasio C, Balestrieri ML, D'Onofrio N. Micro(nano)plastics: an Emerging Burden for Human Health. Int J Biol Sci. 2024 Oct 21;20(14):5779-5792. doi: 10.7150/ijbs.99556. PMID: 39494332; PMCID: PMC11528458.

[82] Kabir ER, Rahman MS, Rahman I. A review on endocrine disruptors and their possible impacts on human health. Environ Toxicol Pharmacol. 2015 Jul;40(1):241-58. doi: 10.1016/j.etap.2015.06.009. Epub 2015 Jun 9. PMID: 26164742.

[83] Alagan M, Chandra Kishore S, Perumal S, Manoj D, Raji A, Kumar RS, Almansour AI, Lee YR. Narrative of hazardous chemicals in water: Its potential removal approach and health effects. Chemosphere. 2023 Sep;335:139178. doi: 10.1016/j.chemosphere.2023.139178. Epub 2023 Jun 9. PMID: 37302496.

[84] Wan MLY, Co VA, El-Nezami H. Endocrine disrupting chemicals and breast cancer: a systematic review of epidemiological studies. Crit Rev Food Sci Nutr. 2022;62(24):6549-6576. doi: 10.1080/10408398.2021.1903382. Epub 2021 Apr 5. PMID: 33819127.

NOTES

◆◇◆

Notes

www.ingramcontent.com/pod-product-compliance
Lightning Source LLC
Chambersburg PA
CBHW032053020426
42335CB00011B/324